The Hauntology of Everyday Life

"Building an arc from Freud's *The Psychopathology of Everyday Life* via Lacan, Winnicott and Derrida to *The Hauntology of Everyday Life,* Rahimi lucidly traces the trajectories through which hauntings have become the hallmark of today's hyper-mediated world. Highlighting a consequential shift from the spectacular violence of traumatic events to the slow structural violence of today's mediascapes in which networked subjectivities are haunted by ghosts in the machine, he introduces his readers to emergent spectral cyberworlds in which "deep fakes in swarming circulation" host ghosts and revenants whose capacities reach far beyond the human senses. In the shadow of AI, however, digital activisms emerge that harness the powers of ghosts for the decolonization of haunted minds and everyday worlds."

—Gabriele Schwab, PhD, Distinguished Professor, *Department of Comparative Literature and Anthropology, University of California, Irvine*

"The Hauntology of Everyday Life is an original, insightful, and timely inquiry into the spectrality of presence. Combining insightful philosophical, cultural, and anthropological reflections with an engrossing psychoanalytic account of Jacques Lacan's theory of trauma, Sadeq Rahimi has written an intelligent meditation on hauntological thinking that enriches our understanding of ghosts in lived experience, historical memory, the social world, and justice."

—Marita Vyrgioti, Associate Lecturer, *University of East London*

"Sadeq Rahimi offers us a remarkably documented text that demonstrates an impressive culture. His reflection around Hauntology is situated at the crossroad between psychoanalysis and philosophy. In dialogue with Lacan, he takes up the idea that a lack is inherent in desire and inscribes it in a broader theorisation: desire as well as words and language, personal and collective representations are haunted by a lack, an unreachable primitive signifier in quest for presentation. This introduces a kind of "worryness" in our relationship to reality, including the very notion of Justice. At the same time, such a worry translates into an ethical responsibility inviting to pay attention to the first signifiers haunting us and to lost voices. Such an approach raises an original and important lighting on a world to become. This complex text is presented in a pedagogical mode that renders our navigation easy and inviting."

—Ellen Corin, PhD, Psychoanalyst and Scientific Secretary, the Montreal Psychoanalytic Society, Emeritus Researcher and Professor in Psychiatry and Anthropology, *McGill University*

The everyday life is full of ghosts, which means full of *petit objet a*, full of *emanet*, full of *La Chose*, *das Ding*, things-in-themselves that are not things at all, but the haunting of their desire and the experience of their absence. Their assemblage constitutes the *hauntology of everyday life*, Sadeq Rahimi argues in this elegantly haunting volume. Reading the intergenerational transmission of affect as constitutive of hauntology, Rahimi presents the complicated and dense texture of memory by anchoring it in specific phantoms of the everyday—a half pack of cigarettes and a ten-Franc coin, given as objects and claimed as *mana*, in words given as things and claimed as ghosts, in the crypt of everyday language that constantly transfers presence to and through absence, in the virtual subjectivities of the present and the haunting presence of the pantemporal (war, colonialism, hunger, genocide, slavery). "What haunts is not that which is gone, it is that which was expected to come but whose condition of arrival has been foreclosed, and the ghost is an advocate of the promised future that was unrightfully cancelled when the past was destroyed" Rahimi writes, fixing thus time (and thus being) as a haunted concept. This is a book that reweaves the warp and the weft of structuralism and symbolism by revisiting the trajectories of language theory and psychoanalysis, from Jacobson, Sebeok, Derrida, and Kristeva through Freud, Victor Turner, Lacan, Raymond Williams, and the political project of Protevi. It is a demanding book that rewards the reader with nuanced and careful microreadings of grand theories.

—Neni Panourgia, PhD, Associate Professor, *Institute for Comparative Literature and Society, Columbia University*

Sadeq Rahimi

The Hauntology of Everyday Life

Foreword by Byron J. Good

palgrave
macmillan

Sadeq Rahimi
Massachusetts Institute of Technology
Cambridge, MA, USA

ISBN 978-3-030-78991-6   ISBN 978-3-030-78992-3   (eBook)
https://doi.org/10.1007/978-3-030-78992-3

This Palgrave Pivot imprint is published by the registered company Springer Nature
Switzerland AG.
The registered company address is: Gewerbestrasse 11, 6330 Cham, Switzerland

To the many ghosts, living and dead, who have left their marks on me.
And to the many whose lives my ghost will mark.

LIVING WITH GHOSTS: FOREWORD TO SADEQ RAHIMI, *THE HAUNTOLOGY OF EVERYDAY LIFE*

Anthropologists live with ghosts. Many of us live and work for important periods of our lives in societies and communities in which spirits and ghosts are part of the everyday social world, almost as present as family members and neighbors, colleagues, and friends. Our driver in Bali honks his horn for a moment as he passes certain crossroads or groves of trees to show respect to the spirits he senses are there. Once driving at night, our car engine simply stopped; while we checked the carburetor, he spent a moment conveying his apology to a spirit he had offended by failing to give proper acknowledgement. Fifteen minutes later we were on our way. A Javanese friend, sleeping in a house we rented in Bali for a few weeks, was troubled at night, until he enlisted Balinese friends in making an offering to the spirit that had been keeping him awake. A man in a village in Java where our friends live sold a piece of his land for a cell phone tower. Not long after, he went mad, being haunted by the spirit of the land he sold without proper permission. My Javanese "god daughter" was lured into marriage by an East Javanese man through love magic, her father believes, and kept her in a violent domestic relationship by continuing to carry out magical rituals, until her father finally enlisted a healer to help free her. A physician friend was troubled by stones being thrown onto his roof at night. Thinking they were being thrown by neighborhood youth, he sent his night watch staff out to find who was doing it, only to learn that no one was there, though the stone throwing continued. He called in a Javanese paranormal, who told him his land was once a Chinese graveyard, and the ghosts were troubling him. The paranormal made offerings, and only then did things become quiet. A *kiyayi*, head of an Islamic residential school or *pesantren*, tells us how when he began clearing the bamboo along the river to make space to develop his school, he would hear the spirits crying at night. The spirits, he told us, use this river as a highway to pass back and forth from Mount Merapi, the sacred volcano north of Yogyakarta, down to the sea to the south, where Nyi Roro Kidul, the great Queen of the South Sea, resides. And so it goes.

Spirits, ghosts, and hauntings are part of everyday life in central Java, where we have lived part-time and worked for the past 25 years. It is through this lens, that of an anthropologist of Indonesia, that I read this manuscript by Sadeq Rahimi on the hauntology of the everyday. It is also through the lens of a friend and longtime collaborator in thinking through the place of hauntology in anthropology, particularly psychological anthropology (see Rahimi & Good, 2019). What is the place of hauntology as a conceptual and interpretive construct for anthropology? Should hauntology be focused on historical trauma and the politicization of memory? What is special about hauntology in contexts in which ghosts and spirits are a part of everyday life? How should anthropologists position themselves within local discourses of haunting ghosts? How do we theorize the "subject" for whom haunting is a reality? Why and how is it that at certain moments in the lives of individuals and societies there seems to be an eruption of ghosts and haunting? And how do we understand responses to such hauntings? This essay represents Sadeq's formulation of the grounds from which questions such as these might be addressed.

Long-standing forms of engagement with the spirit world, as well as new and innovative forms, are as much a part of contemporary modernity in Southeast Asia—and in many parts of the world—as are high-tech medical care and science and engineering, forms of entrepreneurial capitalism, contested legal practices, or constantly evolving religious activities. Encounters with the spirit world may be deadly serious. At the same time, playful engagements with the local world of ghosts and hauntings are key domains of contemporary popular culture and cinema, certainly in Indonesia and Thailand.[1] *Pocong*, ghosts/corpses wrapped in white shrouds that have mistakenly remained "tied" at burial, so that the spirits remain captured rather than freed at burial and float about threateningly, are standard figures in the most popular genre of Indonesian cinema. They are also, quite often, vividly present in the hallucinations of those Javanese suffering psychotic illnesses whom my colleagues and I have come to know. And when Javanese urban *kampung* or neighborhoods charged with COVID-19 control were closed to persons wishing to enter or leave, streets entering the *kampungs* were often guarded by young men dressed as *pocong*. *Pocong* are thus present as realities in everyday life and popular culture, as well as in the direct experiences of those open to that part of the world partially hidden but known to be present.

It is not surprising that spirits, ghosts, and haunting are common sources of ethnographic writing in Southeast Asia. It is surprising, however, that analyses drawing on the writings on hauntology remain relatively absent in anthropology until the last few years. Since the publication of Derrida's *Specters of Marx* (1993, 1994 in English translation), hauntology has been a key analytic project within cultural studies—indeed, so central that in 2013 María del Pilar Blanco and Esther Peeren drew together a large anthology of essays, published between 1999 and 2011, as *The Spectralities Reader: Ghosts and Haunting in Contemporary Cultural Theory*. In the Introduction to the volume, the editors pose the central question of "how, at the end of the twentieth century, a specific metamorphosis occurred of ghosts and haunting from possible actual entities, plot devices, and clichés of common parlance ... into influential conceptual metaphors permeating global (popular) culture and academia alike" (p. 1). This metamorphosis, they note, was signaled by the "sudden preference expressed in 1990s cultural criticism for the somewhat archaic terms 'specter' and 'spectrality' over the mundane 'ghost' and 'ghostliness'" (pp. 1–2). While acknowledging publication of *Specters of Marx* as being the catalyst for what some have called the "spectral turn," they describe the broader influences leading to this theoretical "metamorphosis"—the crucial role of "trauma studies," the larger Derridean corpus and the emergence of deconstruction within literary criticism, as well as graphic and photographic arts in which spectrality is a critical conceptual dimension. Representative essays that emerged within cultural studies from this period are drawn together under headings such as "The Spectral Turn," "Spectropolitics," "Spectral Media," and "Haunted Historiographies."

While "spectrality" framed a large body of writing in cultural studies and literary criticism, "trauma" and "haunting" have been key terms among anthropologists in the emergence of what Derrida called for under the rubric of *hauntology*. Not surprisingly, given the ubiquity of settings of conflict and unspeakable violence, newer generations of anthropologist have increasingly found themselves working in what Michael Fischer (1991) has called "post-trauma politics." Anthropological writing in which "haunting" figures prominently includes writing about societies in which a past history of violence seems to haunt the present in powerful ways, as well as work undertaken in settings of recent or on-going conflict. While images of haunting have long figured in writing about colonialism (Good, Good, and Grayman, 2010), a more recent body of work has focused on "historical trauma" within indigenous societies, where the traces of violence of settler colonialism remain powerful. Explicit use of the powerful metaphors of ghosts and haunting, linking the work directly or indirectly to Derrida and classic works in hauntology, is found in titles such as *Ghosts of War in Vietnam* (Kwon, 2008), *War and Shadows: The Haunting of Vietnam* (Gustafsson, 2009), *Haunting the Korean Diaspora: Shame, Secrecy, and the Forgotten War* (Cho, 2008), *Seeing Like a Child: Inheriting the Korean War* (Han, 2021), and *Ghosts of the New City: Spirits, Urbanity, and the Ruins of Progress in Chiang Mai* (Johnson, 2014).

Other anthropological writing on haunting and hauntology has grown out of ethnographers' experiences working in conflict or post-conflict settings or amidst unthinkable natural disasters. Certainly, that is true of my own work, referenced by Sadeq in the Acknowledgements to this text. In 2005, following the Great Indian Ocean Tsunami that killed nearly 200,000 persons along the coasts of the Indonesian province of Aceh, on the northern tip of Sumatra, my wife Prof. Mary-Jo Good and I began collaborating with the International Organization for Migration (IOM) in developing mental health responses for communities of survivors. As we write elsewhere, the great influx of humanitarian organizations in response to the tsunami quickly faced the complexity of an on-going military conflict between the Free Aceh Movement and the Indonesian military.[2] Though my initial use of the term haunting was in a presentation written immediately after a trip to begin working on a post-conflict project with IOM, which I titled "Haunted by Aceh," my real commitment to making hauntology a central concept in psychological anthropology grew out of the next several years working directly in the field with persons who had experienced horrifying violence from the Indonesian special forces (see Good, 2015). There is something deeply disturbing about listening to intense stories of interrogation and torture, challenging one to ask quite fundamental questions about human nature. Ghosts there were—we heard explicit stories about dreamtime visits of those killed in the tsunami or the conflict. But haunting was present in the on-going experiences of those who had deeply troubling intrusive memories of violence and torture witnessed or experienced personally, memories that would come over and again, day and night, and experienced in the present tense. Our own

others. A brief example is provided from the author's previous wri
schizophrenia in Turkey. And the text points forward to analyses '
of how subjectivity may evolve in relation to "the transition of sociaı aɪ..
personal interactions from the arena of physical presence to the domain of
virtual presence and virtual interactions."

This is a major effort to construct a theoretical framework for addressing the "hauntology of everyday life." It is clearly intended as a foundation
for a longer trajectory of theory-building. I commend it to the readers and
look forward to the conversations it provokes.

Cambridge, MA, USA   Byron J. Good
May 10, 2021

NOTES

1. See Steedly (2013) for an analysis of Indonesian filmic representations of
   ghosts and haunting. Cf. Good and Good (2020) for a commentary.
2. For our work on Aceh, see Good (2015, 2019), Good and Good (2017),
   Good, Grayman, and Good (2016), and Good, Good, and Grayman (2010).

REFERENCES

Abraham, N., & Torok, M. (2005). *The Wolf Man's Magic Word: A Cryptonymy*.
University of Minnesota Press.
Cho, G. M. (2008). *Haunting the Korean Diaspora: Shame, Secrecy, and the
Forgotten War*. University of Minnesota Press.
Del Pilar Blanco, M., & Peeren, E. (Eds.). (2013). *The Spectralities Reader: Ghosts
and Haunting in Contemporary Cultural Theory*. Bloomsbury.
Derrida, J. (1994). *Specters of Marx: The State of the Debt, the Work of Mourning,
and the New International*. Trans. P. Kamuf. Routledge.
Fischer, M. M. J. (1991). Anthropology as Cultural Critique: Inserts for the
1990s. Cultural Studies of Science, Visual-Virtual Realities, and Post-Trauma
Politics. *Cultural Anthropology, 6*, 525–537.
Good, B. J. (2015). Haunted by Aceh: Specters of Violence in Post-Suharto
Indonesia. In D. E. Hinton & A. L. Hinton (Eds.), *Genocide and Mass Violence:
Memory, Symptom, and Recovery* (pp. 58–82). Cambridge University Press.

Good, B. J. (2019). Hauntology: Theorizing the Spectral in Psychological Anthropology. *Ethos, 47*(4), 411–426.

Good, B. J., & Good, M.-J. D. (1994). In the Subjunctive Mode: Epilepsy Narratives in Turkey. *Social Science and Medicine, 38*(6), 835–842.

Good, B., & Good, M.-J. D. (2017). Toward a Cultural Psychology of Trauma and Trauma-Related Disorders. In J. Cassaniti & U. Menon (Eds.), *Universalism Without Uniformity: Exploration in Mind and Culture* (pp. 260–279). Chicago: University of Chicago Press.

Good, B. J., & Good, M.-J. D. (2020). Haunting. *Indonesia* (Special Issues Devoted to Mary Steedly), *109*, 91–97.

Good, M.-J. D., Good, B. J., & Grayman, J. H. (2010). Complex Engagements: Responding to Violence in Postconflict Aceh. In D. Fassin & M. Pandolfi (Eds.), *Contemporary States of Emergency: The Politics of Military and Humanitarian Interventions* (pp. 241–266). Zone Books.

Good, B. J., Grayman, J., & Good, M.-J. D. (2016). Is PTSD a 'Good Enough' Concept for Post-Conflict Mental Health Work? Reflections on Work in Aceh, Indonesia. In D. E. Hinton & B. J. Good (Eds.), *Culture and PTSD: Trauma in Global and Historical Perspective* (pp. 387–417). University of Pennsylvania Press.

Gordon, A. F. (2008). *Ghostly Matters: Haunting and the Sociological Imagination.* University of Minnesota Press.

Gustafsson, M. L. (2009). *War and Shadows: The Haunting of Vietnam.* Cornell University Press.

Han, C. (2021). *Seeing Like a Child: Inheriting the Korean War.* Fordham University Press.

Johnson, A. A. (2014). *Ghosts of the New City: Spirits, Urbanity, and the Ruins of Progress in Chiang Mai.* University Hawai'i Press.

Kwon, H. (2008). *Ghosts of War in Vietnam.* Cambridge University Press.

Lincoln, M., & Lincoln, B. (2015). Toward a Critical Hauntology: Bare Afterlife and the Ghosts of Ba Chúc. *Comparative Studies in Society and History, 57*, 191–220.

Rahimi, S., & Good, B. J. (2019). Preface: Ghosts, haunting, and hauntology. *Ethos, 47*(4), 409–410.

Steedly, M. M. (2013). Transparency and Apparition: Media Ghosts of Post-New Order Indonesia. In P. Spyer & M. M. Steedly (Eds.), *Images that Move* (pp 257–294). School for Advanced Research Press.

ACKNOWLEDGMENTS

Like everything else, every book is first and foremost a palimpsest. And as with every palimpsest, it will always be a futile effort to try and identify all the traces left and faded over time. My interest in ghosts and haunting started long ago in Shiraz, when, as an adolescent in post-revolutionary Iran, I picked up the unusual hobby of hypnotizing friends and relatives, and before long, learned that I could easily turn my hypnotized subjects into mediums channeling various ghosts to speak through their mouths. My cousin Davood was one of my best and most dedicated subjects, and I will not even try to remember all the dead celebrities, ranging from Genghis Khan and Stalin to Jesus, Elvis, and Albert Einstein, who showed up and spoke to me through Davood. The days of seances and spirit channeling eventually came to an end as the original curiosity wore off and gave its place mostly to the fear of the unknown and the misunderstood. But as I sit down decades later to acknowledge my debts, intellectual, and otherwise, for a book on hauntology, it is impossible not to feel grateful to Davood for his transparent love, interest, and generosity which helped graduate my curiosity about ghosts into new questions. Decades later, my interest in ghosts and the spectral was sparked again, this time in New Orleans, where I was invited to present on a panel about the uncanny at the biennial conference of the Society for Psychological Anthropology (SPA). I remain grateful to Sarah Pinto for inviting me to join that panel. It was on that same panel that my dear friend and mentor, Byron J. Good, presented a piece, brief and elegant as ever, but which carried in it something different: an unspoken trace of trauma. Byron had just returned from fieldwork in Aceh, and his talk was aptly titled "Haunted by Aceh." I remember very well how what he communicated that day went well beyond the short text of that talk, or even the cracking voice or the tears in his eyes as he spoke of years of exposure to the aftermaths of multiple waves of trauma in Aceh ranging from decades of savage warfare, large-scale murders, and widespread torture, to tsunamis and earthquakes. He was genuinely haunted, even if by proxy, and his talk brought the notion of haunting into strong resonance with my own findings at the time about how closely the experience of the uncanny is tied to the fundamental processes of ego formation. I was teaching cultural psychiatry and psychological anthropology in Canada at the time, and it did not take long after returning from New Orleans that I submitted my first ethics application for a research project on ghosts and haunting. And the rest is history, as they say. But Byron Good has continued to be a source of inspiration and a wonderful colleague to dialogue with about ghosts and haunting in all these years. We have had a number of seminars and conferences on haunting and hauntology together since New Orleans, including day-long conferences at Harvard and elsewhere, double-panels at SPA, graduate courses on hauntology and postcolonial disorders, and last year (2020) we co-edited a special issue of *Ethos* dedicated to haunting and hauntology. My gratitude to Byron is tremendous and on-going. I would be remiss, however, if I did not mention Ellen Corin, another substantial mentor and friend and one of the most inspiring psychoanalysts I have known, whose ideas have long inspired and guided me. Ellen's beautiful way of thinking about subjectivity and haunting, which is simultaneously poetic, clinical, and academic, has been a generous source of learning for me. Michael M.J. Fischer, who has also been so kind to agree to write an epilogue to this volume, has long been another source of brilliant inspiration for me. Mike's awe-inspiringly vast and deep knowledge covers so much that regardless of what topic I need to think about, he is always one of the first people whose thoughts on the topic I want to hear. And finally, I left my sons Reza and Kianoush for last, because to them goes my most special gratitude and love. I am so grateful to Aatash Reza, who so generously spent hours audio recording books and papers on hauntology in his warm and professional voice, so that I can have the luxury of listening to them on my walks or while driving. And I am deeply grateful to Kianoush, who paid such close attention and care to this book project and to me working my way through it. He put so much love into motivating and pushing me to write at moments when I did not feel like writing, and made sure that I met my deadlines like I should. Without his caring, this book may not have been!

CONTENTS

CHAPTER 1

A Hauntology for Everyday Life

Abstract This chapter outlines the basic objectives of the book and highlights the general theoretical grounds on which the book develops its central argument that all human experience is fundamentally haunted. The primary points of reference include psychoanalytic theory, specifically Jacques Lacan's object relational theory of ego development and his reading and expansion of Freud's theory of the psychic apparatus and its dynamics; along with the Hegelian ontology of the negative and its later modifications by twentieth-century philosophers such as Heidegger and Derrida; and the semiotics of difference introduced by Saussure and worked by Jakobson and others. Whereas ontology can be read as an attempt to exorcise "reality as such" from the ambiguities that irreducibly haunt human experience of reality, hauntology is described here as an evocation that seeks not to exorcise, but simply to recognize and address the endless ghosts that are created by the very act of human perception and cognition, and hence subjective experience. Finally, hauntology is outlined here as a mode of understanding power and its working in ways fundamentally different from historical, archaeological, or even a Foucauldian genealogical modality, in that instead of attempting to establish that which was, hauntological analysis seeks to recognize—to allow to come forward, to speak—that which had been to be but was not, that which could have been, the future that hailed the past but was forced to disappear from its horizon.

Keywords Hauntology • Ontology • Ghosts • Exorcism • Subjectivity • Psychoanalysis • Semiotics, Philosophy • Presence

> *I reimagine my haunting spirit not as an omnipotent God but as a weak force, a quiet call, an invitation, a solicitation. This God is not a "necessary being" but a "maybe," a "perhaps," whose "might" is the subjunctive might of the might-be it whispers in my ear.*
> —John D. Caputo

When Sigmund Freud published *The Psychopathology of Everyday Life* in 1907, he opted to open it with a two-line epigraph drawn from Goethe's *Faust* which, in first glance, strikes one as strangely irrelevant to the book's basic topic. "Now," says Faust, "the air is so filled with ghosts / that no one knows how to escape them" (Part II, Act V, Scene 5).[1] Freud was famously particular with his words, and still more so with his openings. So why then, one might ask, would he choose to start a book about the everyday life with a statement about ghosts filling the air? It is my intention through this book to make it clear how Freud's reference to an air filled with spooks is not only not irrelevant, but in fact about the most appropriate epigraph he could have chosen to open a book about the fundamental processes of the human psychic apparatus.

Often identified as one of Freud's most widely read and translated books, *The Psychopathology of Everyday Life* is dedicated to driving home one basic idea: that a close study of the daily mental processes, specifically slips and failures of the human mind, reveals that dreams and waking time perceptions are governed by the same set of psychic processes. Freud then uses this understanding to reach the foundational conclusion that the boundary between the "normal" and "abnormal" states of subjectivity is unclear, unstable, and as such, nonexistent. This is one of the most substantial contributions among Freud's extraordinary array of ideas. The notion of neuroticism, which is by far the hallmark of psychoanalytic thought, is entirely dependent on this reading, as are such notions as transference or the associative structure of psychic processes and hence the very possibility of psychoanalysis as the "talking cure."

But still, why would Freud open a book about the most foundational features of "the psychic apparatus" with the image of a space so saturated with ghosts that no one can avoid them? To be bold, the answer is because ghosts and haunting are so central to Freud's work that he could not avoid them, just as I could not avoid naming or starting this book with the mention of Freud's work.[2] What *The Hauntology of Everyday Life* is meant to put forward is that the very space of everyday life is so filled with ghosts that nobody can avoid them—in fact, that the very experience of everyday life is built around a process that we can call hauntogenic, and whose major by-product is a steady stream of ghosts.

One of the challenging revelations that the latter half of the twentieth-century psychoanalytic theory had to deal with was due to the impressive novel ideas that French psychoanalyst Jacques Lacan managed to "pull" out of Freud's texts. Ideas that had apparently laid dormant inside Freud's text for decades now came out in ways that were simultaneously impossible to reject and troublesome to reconcile with the official canon that was already built over Freud's tomb. Around the same time, another French philosopher, Jacques Derrida, was mapping his own rebellion, a map that while clearly distinct from Lacan's work, feels impressively "of the same material," if nothing else due to the fact that three major intellectual streams: Freudian psychoanalysis of the unconscious, Hegelian metaphysics of the spirit, and Saussurean semiotics of difference, saturate the warp and weft of both textures. Much has been said and written on similarities and differences between Lacan and Derrida, and it would be of little benefit to repeat that here. It would be sufficient for my purposes here to simply point out the common moment in which they thought and spoke, the shared intellectual Geist that informed their ideations, despite the many ways in which they aimed their thoughts toward distinct desired ends.

In order to argue for hauntology as the appropriate language for speaking of basic human experiences, one may think of a few layers of significance. At the very core of these so-called layers would be meaning and its formation, which is so closely entangled with the formation of desire as to be considered one and the same. This core duo sets the foundation of the range of human subjective experiences including thought, speech, textuality, and temporality, along with drive, affect, power, and politicality. The ensemble of these effects translates in turn into what we identify as the domain of ontology, and its subsidiary, epistemology. Simply put, the call to hauntological thinking entails the call to a fundamentally different mode of understanding the human subject, including what makes it tick, what drives it, and what the nature of its experienced reality is. The difference is in fact so extensive as to offer a way to think about subjectivity without a subject and free from an androcentric bias. This possibility promises a new theoretic frame of reference capable of accommodating virtual or networked subjectivity as the outcome of predominantly online human-human and human-machine interactions, socializations, and collaborations. If so, then a hauntological theory of subjectivity may also offer the suitable conceptual framework for thinking about artificial subjectivity—synthetic subjectivity without human agency. I hope to briefly address this question in the final sections of this volume, but I intend to tackle it more extensively in my upcoming volume on the notion of networked subjectivity.

"Let us call it a hauntology," says Derrida, "this logic of haunting would not be merely larger and more powerful than an ontology or a thinking of Being...It would harbor within itself, but like circumscribed places or particular effects, eschatology and teleology themselves."[3] Hauntology does not ask, "to be or not to be"; it claims instead the simultaneous playfulness of "to be and not to be." Hauntology is always subjunctive, to go back to John Caputo's poetic notion of God's subjunctive might,[4] or to Byron and Mary-Jo Good's ethnographic discovery of a "subjunctive world, one in which healing is an open possibility, even if miracles are necessary."[5] Hauntology may be understood as an act of reading informed by the fact that the word is the death of the thing, as Hegel emphasized. The word comes to be only after the death of the thing, yet it is not the death of the thing that renders the word meaningful. The word is a word only insofar as it is haunted by the spectral presence of the dead thing—and other dead words. If the word is haunted, then the act of reading can take two basic postures toward the text: as hauntology, or as exorcism. There are of course different modalities of exorcism, as in one that seeks to extract and conjure away a ghost that is deemed destructive, polluting, pathogenic, or in any case *unwanted*; and another that seeks to liberate, vindicate, revive, or in any case *help* the ghost leave the confinements of a haunted place, person, society, or text. But whether sympathetic or antithetical, while a hauntological reading would strive to admit the presence of the ghost and seeks to unearth and unpack to the extent possible a text's layers and dynamics of spectral presences, an exorcism, whether benign or aggressively postured, intends and attempts to separate, to identify, to recover and release one or the other (the haunted, or the haunter) by extracting and naming the ghost that haunts.

When hauntological reading is performed successfully, it manages to animate a text/subject through an outpouring of ghosts and other spectral entities from the otherwise silent depths of the text/psyche. In

from any political allegiance or moral point of reference beyond the sub
sively simple idea of acknowledging the presence of the absents, and hear-
ing the voices of the silenced. But what could possibly be more impactful,
politically impactful, than to understand and unpack the present for what it
is and for all that it is? In order to select strategic social or political lines of
move, or to design effective interventions, we need to first understand the
possibilities, hopes and desires that were once and are no longer available
to the public conscious, to unearth and exhume crypts in which suppressed
dreams of past communities and their lost moments are trapped. This is
clearly a different strategy from history, from archaeology, and even from a
Foucauldian genealogy, in that instead of attempting to establish that
which was, hauntological analysis seeks to know—to allow to speak, to be
more specific—that which was to be, that which could have been but never
was, the future that hailed the past but then disappeared from the horizon.
Not a search for the truth, this is a hunt for the non-Truth, for the absent
force whose effect can be seen, but not its source, its shape, its location or
its time even, except in the form of an "imagined" spectrality. "Can we,
should we, try and excavate utopia?" asks Owen Hatherley at the beginning of *Militant Modernism*.[12] And that is perhaps a question that we all
need to be asking, whether we are in the business of excavating and eman-
cipating or simply waiting for utopias to show on the horizon, or in the
work of heeding and warning and seeking to prevent them.

NOTES

1. *Nun ist die Luft von solchem Spuk so voll / Daß niemand weiß wie er ihn meiden soll* (Goethe, 1862).
2. See pp. 17–20 of Mary S. Gossy's (1995) book, *Freudian Slips: Woman, Writing, the Foreign Tongue*, for another interesting account of Freud's epigraph to *The Psychopathology of Everyday Life*.
3. Derrida, 1994, p. 10.
4. Caputo, 2012, p. 33.
5. Good and Good, 1994, p. 839.
6. Derrida, 1994, p. 221.
7. Derrida, 1981, p. 144.
8. Derrida, 1994, p. 202.
9. Derrida, 1994, p. 13.
10. Ibid.
11. Derrida, 1994, p. 202, emphasis mine.
12. Hatherley, 2009, p. 3.

REFERENCES

Caputo, J. D. (2012). Teaching the Event: Deconstruction, Hauntology, and the Scene of Pedagogy. In C. W. Ruitenberg (Ed.), *Philosophy of Education* (pp. 23–34). Philosophy of Education Society.

Derrida, J. (1981). *Dissemination*. Trans. B. Johnson. Continuum.

Derrida, J. (1994). *Specters of Marx: The State of the Debt, the Work of Mourning, and the New International*. Trans. P. Kamuf. Routledge.

Freud, S. (1901). The Psychopathology of Everyday Life: Forgetting, Slips of the Tongue, Bungled Actions, Superstitions and Errors. In J. Strachey (Ed. & Trans.), *Standard Edition of the Complete Psychological Works of Sigmund Freud* (Vol. VI, pp. VII-296). The Hogarth Press.

Goethe, J. W. (1862). *Faust*. D. Nutt.

Good, B. J., & Good, M.-J. D. (1994). In the Subjunctive Mode: Epilepsy Narratives in Turkey. *Social Science and Medicine, 38*(6), 835–842.

Gossy, M. S. (1995). *Freudian Slips: Woman, Writing, the Foreign Tongue*. University of Michigan Press.

Hatherley, O. (2009). *Militant Modernism*. Zero Books.

CHAPTER 2

Meaning, Language, and Subjectivity

Abstract This chapter focuses on the core idea that the production of meaning is a hauntogenic event, as the process that creates meaning also creates spectral traces of the original events and entities that are made sense of. As infants develop they master the creation of symbols to represent sense impressions of external and internal events, entities and experiences; followed by the ability to communicate such representations in the social space of a symbolic system. Through each wave of elevated representation spectral traces of the signified entities and experiences are also produced, silent/negative references to an original object which "haunt" the new signifier. The process of transformation of a "thing in itself" to a signifier is examined here with specific attention to the role played by phonemes, which serve as gateways between somatic and cognitive levels of experience. The discussion continues with an examination of the psychoanalytic notion of Nachträglichkeit. Freud introduced Nachträglichkeit to explain the clinical observation that some old and forgotten events find a way of returning to life to assert traumatic impact, often with more devastating force than did the actual experience. This chapter will serve as the foundation for upcoming discussions of the higher levels of representation, as these semiotic structures make possible the emergence of desire and its psychological economy in tandem with death drive through higher level linguistic functions such as metaphoricity and metonymy.

9

Keywords Semiosis • Hauntogenesis • Phoneme • Representation •
Symbols • Signifiers • Nachträglichkeit • Trauma • das Ding

> *All heart they live, all head, all eye, all ear,*
> *All intellect, all sense, and as they please,*
> *They limb themselves, and colour, shape, or size,*
> *Assume, as likes them best, condense or rare.*
> —John Milton

Hauntology has quickly exploded to become an almost ubiquitous descriptor in certain lines of inquiry, specifically those concerned with the topics of historical memory and trauma. Such dedicated usage introduces at least two challenges: needless to say, it risks fixating the term's conceptual reference within a narrow field of investigation; and perhaps more importantly, the somewhat self-obvious relevance of the term to the fields of history and especially trauma in a somewhat metaphoric sense can lead to a less-than-rigorous attention to the broader mechanisms involved and the genuinely ubiquitous relevance of hauntology to "everyday life." By "broader mechanisms" I am referring primarily to the semiotic and linguistic processes that make possible the very experience of haunting and, due to their foundational status, necessitate a hauntological model of not just subjective experience, but epistemology and in fact ontology as such. I will attempt to outline a semiotic and linguistic discussion of these processes in this and the next chapter respectively, which will hopefully drive home why a hauntological analysis needs to understand "haunting" in terms more detailed than historical or individual events and their specific social or psychological aftermath. To do so, I will discuss the hauntogenic nature of foundational semiotic processes as they translate and deliver sense impressions of events and substances to abstract sensa and perceptual meaning, which in turn make possible the subjective experience of desire and its extensive psychological economy. This formulation provides a core argument for why features of this operation not only set the stage for, but in fact necessitate a hauntological analysis of subjective experience as such. As I will describe in this and the next chapter, it is precisely this hauntogenic process that makes possible the later appearance of *objet a*, the object cause of desire, and the so-called death drive, leading to the formation and emergence of subjective experience as such.

It is now almost a truism to say that human subjectivity, and the very capacity for subjective experience as we know it, are not simply associated with but fundamentally dependent on the capacities of production and processing of meaning, and the presence of a structured symbolic order for the communication of that meaning, language serving as a most immediately observable example. It is, after all, the evolutionary emergence of the ability to create, process, and communicate symbols, and the emergence of an inter-personal structure that guides and orders the communication of such symbols, that marks the basic turning point in the appearance of Homo sapiens and what we understand as human social subjectivity. If we were to graph a basic trajectory tracing the progression of solid, lifeless matter to the human subject in its social and symbolic complexity, we can simply plot a graph with time on one axis, and abstraction as the other.[1] The evolutionary process that has led to the contemporary state of human subjectivity, in other words, can be traced in terms of a consecutive set of elevations in abstract representation and the means of communicating the resulting information. I don't intend to engage the broad question of abstraction as an evolutionary development, but the developmental process of abstraction, which also holds a foundational place in current theories of human development,[2] offers important concepts for a hauntological model of subjectivity which we need to understand. Consider the basic process through which internal physical and chemical experiences are abstracted and merge with the collectively maintained systems of meanings to produce thoughts and emotions, for instance. Psychoanalytic thought over the past century has developed a solid array of concepts for examination of this process, laid originally by Freud and later refined and expanded by Lacan.

PHONEMES AND THINGS

The concept of *das Ding*, "the Thing," is one such concept around which to set up this discussion, even if, ironically enough, the most accurate description of the Thing might be that which is a no-thing. As we will see in this chapter, this adds a whole new level of meaning to the basic definition of language as a means of communicating that which is absent. The "absent" in this sense goes well beyond the absent sun about which I can use language to tell stories at night. This sense of absent refers to the idea that language as such is the result and the manifestation of a fundamental absence: the absence of the self to itself. The so-called signifier, that is to say, is the vehicle, a signifier, of a thing that is absent not just in the physical or even phenomenological sense of absence, but in the ontological sense of an absent "something" that cannot be signified and yet whose absence can only be experienced through the act of signification. The signifier serves to mark an imagined location dedicated to that unknown (unknown insofar as it cannot be signified and made sense of) which is sought. The core, in other words, around which I have just proposed to cast the hauntological understanding of language and meaning, is a hollow one. This is of course not my innovation: "through the word, which is already a presence made of absence," says Lacan, "absence itself comes to have a name."[3] As frustratingly vacuous and circular as what I have just outlined may seem, through another well-established tradition, the work of Hegel may be able to help better understand this central piece of the puzzle. Specifically, consider Hegel's elaboration of the process whereby the thing "in itself" (*an sich*) is elevated to the "for itself" (*für sich*).

In a passage in his *Encyclopedia*,[4] where Hegel elaborates the progression from abstracted imagination to thought, he offers an analysis of the process through which a "thing," that is, a thing as it is in itself, becomes an object—object of understanding to a human subject. "The name," he says, is "the thing so far as it exists and counts in the ideational realm."[5] As a "thing in itself" is transformed to, or rather replaced by, an "object" within the "ideational realm," the new object, which is now identified with "word", is simultaneously "the death of the thing," while retaining nonetheless a certain relation with the thing. To borrow from Heidegger reading Kant: "Kant does explicitly distinguish between the thing as an appearance (*Erscheinung*) and as thing-in-itself (*Ding an sich*). But the thing-in-itself, i.e., detached from and taken out of every relation of manifestation for us, remains for us a mere x [and] in every thing as an appearance we unavoidably think also of this x."[6] Even if the hark back to this unknown "x" may be inevitable, that does not necessitate an awareness of such relation by the subject—this is a spectral relation, as Derrida would later describe it. And to be sure, "we think in names."[7] In other words, insofar as thought is the dynamic articulation of and the interaction between words (i.e. mental objects), all thought is already haunted by the ghost of the thing. In the words of Maurice Blanchot, "death alone allows me to grasp what I want to attain; it exists in words as the only way they can have meaning."[8]

As compelling as the accounts provided by Hegel—and others—of the transformation of a thing to object/word, or sensa to sense[9] may be, layering in a linguistic/semiotic reading of the process can add substantial, and perhaps more accessible, texture to the psycho-philosophical account. Consider phonemes,[10] for instance, which are generally understood as the basic building block of language, since they are the last identifiable "units" as we unpack what language is made of. "Philosophical terminology," says Jakobson, "tends to call the various sign systems languages, and language properly so-called word language."[11] But, he goes on to add, "it would perhaps be possible to identify it more accurately by calling it phoneme language. This phoneme language is the most important of the various sign systems, it is for us language par excellence, language properly so-called, language *tout court*."[12] And this is so for the basic reason that phonemes are the smallest units of language before you are no longer dealing with "language," before you enter the realm of purely affective and somatic forces, the realm of the "imaginary," in Lacanian jargon. It is this last feature, the borderline location of phonemes, that is of interest to me here, as it establishes the paradoxical character of phonemes, "which simultaneously signify and yet are devoid of all meaning."[13]

Insofar as language consists of a system of signs built on the principle of binary oppositions,[14] phonemes carry the task of laying a broad and finely pixelated groundwork of phonic oppositions that are then used to produce higher level combinations such as graphemes and morphemes or words. Phonemes, said Saussure, are "above all else oppositive, relative and negative entities."[15] This basic feature of phonemes as part physical (sounds) and part symbolic (signs indicating opposition), makes them the ideal mediator between the visceral and the symbolic, both of which realms are also organized in terms of oppositions and associations, albeit in different modalities of organization. While it is sufficiently easy to identify the nature and the role played by oppositions in the physical/acoustic level of phonemes, however, it is somewhat unclear how a relation of association comes to be established between phonemic opposing binaries. As Hegel has elaborated,[16] internal concepts stand in relation to each other through a network of associations that establishes the whole of the psychic/perceptual edifice, in a "relation of necessary implication."[17] Such relation of necessary implication is precisely the modality that Saussure borrowed from Husserl in describing his structural semiotics. Ironically enough, however, Jakobson demonstrates that at the lowest physical stratum of the linguistic sign system, phonemes in fact fail to adhere to this basic structural principle: unlike the broad relation of implication that holds within the psychic apparatus as well as within the linguistic system of signs, he finds it impossible to attribute a self-evident system of relationality beyond oppositionality to phonemes.[18] Rather than simply opening a case of exception for phonemes, however, Jakobson is able to identify a separate set, a set of *phenomenological* oppositions that tie phonemes together in a relation of implication. What makes this surprising find especially relevant for us is that these relations are primarily based on bodily conditions of production/articulation of phonemes, such as the shape of lips, tenseness or laxity of muscles, degree of air pressure, location of articulation (buccal resonator), and so on. In addition to providing a clear system of binaries, in other words, these oppositions highlight the physical and embodied locatedness of phonemes as parts of a whole (a phenomenological gestalt), and thence an associative network of "necessary implications" among them: tenseness is necessarily related to laxness, back of buccal resonator automatically stands in opposition to and in association with its front, and so on. So here we have a clear situation where physical phenomenological experience interfaces and merges with the symbolic meaning system through the "two faced" function of phonemes. I will present a similarly Janusian characteristic later, when examining metaphors as a higher level gateway connecting phenomenological sensa and linguistic sense, as Ricoeur has demonstrated. But what I would like us to take away from Jakobson's discovery concerning this Janusian function of phonemes is the role it plays in the production of language as a symbolic system that is always already "haunted" by the biological, or to bring this back to the psychoanalytic jargon, by *das Ding*.

In short then, here at the level of phonemes we find the opportunity to observe the linguistic and phenomenological roots of a capacity or quality that permeates the edifice of "language" as such, insofar as language is the space where *das Ding* is (re)created. But, while Jakobson's elaborations on sound and meaning give us a clear way of understanding and formulating phonemes and their amphibian performance as the "hinge" around which somatic and semiotic registers are fused together, we still need to layer this further with a psychosemiotic model of the birth of desire and the mechanisms through which individual ego manages to anchor itself within the fluid ocean of meanings, in order to complete a map of the way *das Ding* ends up haunting the sign, the language, and the subject as such. Let us pause here and ponder for a moment as we move into the psychoanalytic discussion, Merleau-Ponty's emphasis that "the philosophy of Freud is not a philosophy of the body, but of the flesh."[19]

NACHTRÄGLICHKEIT

Freud introduced the term *Nachträglichkeit* as he struggled to develop a model for trauma. Specifically, he struggled to conceptualize his own and others' recurrent observation that trauma experienced—or imagined to have been experienced—in distant past may be evoked, or invoked, by specific events, and people may be affected in unexpected ways by traumatic events that seem to have woken and returned from long-forgotten recesses of their history. While it seems to have aroused much interest across other fields, *Nachträglichkeit* has received far less psychoanalytic attention than many of Freud's conceptualizations, a fact in part responsible also for the lack of a standardized translation of the word in literature. *Nachträglichkeit* has been translated into an array of different terms depending on context and usage, such as "latency," "retroactive temporality," "retrospective attribution," "belatedness," "delayed onset trauma," "deferred action," "après-coup," and "afterwardsness".[20] As I mentioned, Freud developed the idea as he struggled to make sense of the observation that many of the cases of "hysteria" seemed to be in fact caused by evocations of old and long-forgotten traumatic events, with the basic model emerging that even a small event could trigger memories of old and forgotten traumatic events, often from childhood, which would now be interpreted and re-experienced in much stronger traumagenic terms by the adult person. An old, dormant if you like, trauma would thus be invoked to life, and while it may not have had much of an impact on the person's mind during its first occurrence, in its second coming it could exert a fully-fledged traumatic impact. It is this second coming and its aftermath that Freud called *Nachträglichkeit*.[21] In Freud's own words, *Nachträglichkeit* is the process "of a memory arousing an affect which it did not arouse as an experience, because in the meantime the change [from the early self that experienced the event to the current one that remembers it] had made possible a different understanding of what was remembered."[22] The temporal dislocation of an experience (or of its impact, to be precise) is the central piece in this formulation—in order for the nature and aftermath of a past event to change in the present, the past has to be present in some sense. The second important point here, at least for our discussion, is the notion of the "missed" or the lacking meaning, the part of the event that fails to be translated into "understanding" at the time of the event, and which can come back later in time to possess the subject's psyche—but only when the subject is capable of processing and cogitating that missing part into the symbolic order of meaning, and hence experiencing it in new terms.

You may have noted that this missed part, this left out "thing" is in many ways reminiscent of the idea of *das Ding*, the part of the actual experienced event or sensed thing that fails to make it to the mental or linguistic object and which "stays back" to lurk somewhere below the symbolic register. The "traumatic" event in fact has remained a non-event because the traumagenic elements have remained outside the subject's domain of symbolic interpretation/understanding. As a result the event is not in a position to effect any consequences—not until a version of the subject comes along that is capable of recognizing and decoding the missing eventuality of the event, and channels the dormant event into the realm of meaning and consequences, and hence gives it the voice to claim and demand a consequence using its newly-gained power as a legitimate part of the symbolic order. In his work, Jean Laplanche has conceptualized this same notion in the form of a question, an unanswerable question, that a child picks up early in life, but which they may never find an answer to. Laplanche borrows Lacan's terms to call the so-called question an enigmatic signifier, which is passed on to the child by adults through what he describes as a "primal seduction," and thenceforth serves to intrigue and motivate the child's psychic development as they undertake a quest to arrive at the missing meaning.[23] I don't intend to enter a closer reading of Laplanche here, but simply to point out the obvious point in his account, namely the significant developmental role played by a missing something as we grow and learn to transform/translate physical experiences and phenomenological sensa to the realm of mental objects, cognitive representations, and linguistic sense.

The Thing, *das Ding*, is a part of what is sensed and subsequently transformed from pure materiality to abstracted (prelinguistic) perception which fails to "make it" through such transformation and thus remains associated with the abstracted image (if we can call it that) in the form of an unconscious reference. Now, *das Ding*, however, is only half way through the process of symbolic representation.

NOTES

1. See for instance the works of Jakob von Uexküll (e.g. Von Uexküll, 2013); Thomas Sebeok (e.g. Sebeok, 2001); or Kalevi Kull (e.g. Kull, 1999; Kull et al., 2011).
2. E.g. Piaget, 2014; Sigel, 2013.

3. Lacan, 1953, p. 228.
4. Hegel, 1975.
5. Hegel, 1975, p. 219.
6. Heidegger, 1967, p. 128.
7. Hegel, 1975, p. 220.
8. Blanchot, 1981, p. 43.
9. See Ricoeur, 2003. I will reintroduce this connection later in discussing metaphoricity.
10. "Phonic elements by means of which words are differentiated [but] have no positive and fixed meaning of their own." (Jakobson, 1978, p. 69)
11. Jakobson, 1978, p. 67.
12. Ibid.
13. Ibid.
14. See Saussure, 1959.
15. Quoted in Jakobson 1978, p. 76.
16. Hegel (1975), see also Boothby (2001) for a detailed elaboration of this theme.
17. "If one of the terms is given, then the other, though not present, is evoked" (Jakobson, 1978, p. 76).
18. See e.g. Jakobson 1978, pp. 76ff.
19. Merleau-Ponty, 1968, p. 270.
20. Eickhoff, 2006.
21. See for instance Freud 1894, 1895, 1896 for earlier development of the term. His earliest use of the term has been traced to his letters to Fliess, he used the notion quite often through his later works. See Laplanche, 2005, pp. 377–79.
22. Freud, 1895, p. 356. See case of Emma.
23. See e.g. Laplanche, 1999.

References

Blanchot, M. (1981) *"Literature and the Right to Death," "The Gaze of Orpheus" and Other Literary Essays.* Trans. L. Davis, ed. P. A. Sitney. Station Hill Press.

Boothby, R. (2001). *Freud as Philosopher: Metapsychology After Lacan.* Psychology Press.

Eickhoff, F.-W. (2006). On *Nachträglichkeit:* The Modernity of an Old Concept. *International Journal of Psychoanalysis, 87,* 1453–1469.

Freud, S. (1894). The Neuro-Psychoses of Defense. In J. Strachey (Ed. & Trans.), *Standard Edition of the Complete Psychological Works of Sigmund Freud* (Vol. III, pp. 45–61). The Hogarth Press.

Freud, S. (1895). Project for a Scientific Psychology. In J. Strachey (Ed. & Trans.), *Standard Edition of the Complete Psychological Works of Sigmund Freud* (Vol. I, pp. 281–397). The Hogarth Press.

Freud, S. (1896). Further Remarks on the Neuro-Psychoses of Defense. In J. Strachey (Ed. & Trans.), *Standard Edition of the Complete Psychological Works of Sigmund Freud* (Vol. III, pp. 162–185). The Hogarth Press.

Hegel, G. W. F. (1975). *Logic, Being Part One of the Encyclopedia of the Philosophical Sciences*. Trans. W. Wallace. Clarendon Press.

Heidegger, M. (1967). *What Is a Thing?* Trans. W. B. Barton Jr. and V. Deutsch. Gateway Editions.

Jakobson, R. (1978). *Six Lectures on Sound and Meaning*. Trans. J. Mepham. MIT Press.

Kull, K. (1999). Biosemiotics in the Twentieth Century: A View from Biology. *Semiotica, 127*(1–4), 385–414.

Kull, K., Deacon, T., Emmeche, C., Hoffmeyer, J., & Stjernfelt, F. (2011). Theses on Biosemiotics: Prolegomena to a Theoretical Biology. In *Towards a Semiotic Biology: Life Is the Action of Signs* (pp. 25–41). World Scientific Publishing/ Imperial College Press.

Lacan, J. (1953/1996). The function and field of speech and language in psychoanalysis. In J. Lacan, *Ecrits: The First Complete Edition in English*, Trans. B. Fink, H. Fink and R. Grigg. New York: W. W. Norton & Company, 197–268.

Laplanche, J. (1999). *Essays on Otherness*. Routledge.

Laplanche, J. (2005). Deferred Action. In A. D. E. Mijolla (Ed.), *International Dictionary of Psychoanalysis* (pp. 377–380). Macmillan.

Merleau-Ponty, M. (1968). *The Visible and the Invisible*. Trans. A. Lingis. Northwestern University Press.

Piaget, J. (2014). *Studies in Reflecting Abstraction*. Psychology Press.

Ricoeur, P. (2003). *The Rule of Metaphor*. Routledge.

Saussure, F. D. (1959). *Course in General Linguistics*. Trans. W. Baskin. Philosophical Library.

Sebeok, T. A. (2001). *Global semiotics*. Indiana University Press.

Sigel, I. E. (Ed.). (2013). *Development of Mental Representation: Theories and Applications*. Psychology Press.

Von Uexküll, J. (2013). *A Foray into the Worlds of Animals and Humans: With a Theory of Meaning* (Vol. 12). University of Minnesota Press.

CHAPTER 3

Ghosts, Metaphors, and Structures of Feeling

Abstract This chapter builds on and expands the earlier discussion of haunted nature of meaning, as physical reality is translated into symbolic meaning, focusing on higher-level processes of linguistic communication and subjective experience, such as the metaphoric and metonymic modalities of language, intersubjective and intergenerational transmission of affective patterns. I draw on the theoretic discussions including the notion of hauntology advanced by Jacques Derrida, structures of feeling outlined by Raymond Williams, phantoms and cryptonymy by Nicolas Abraham and Maria Torok, along with Freudian, Object Relational, and Lacanian psychoanalytic models of ego formation to drive home the fundamental role played by the negativity (the lack of the Thing) which, as discussed in the last chapter, is introduced into the very structure of consciousness from the earliest stages of production of meaning. This chapter also discusses the pantemporality of subjective experience and the relationship of this fact to the hauntological nature of meaning, and the phenomenon of death drive postulated by Freud. The chapter ends with a discussion of political subjectivity and the implications of hauntological theory of experience for social and generational transmission of patterns of political affect, as well as a brief examination of the relevance of this

An earlier version of this chapter has been published in the journal *Subjectivity* (see Rahimi, 2016)

S. Rahimi, *The Hauntology of Everyday Life*,
https://doi.org/10.1007/978-3-030-78992-3_3

conceptualization for emerging modalities of subjectivity, including net-worked human subjectivity or the possibility of artificial subjectivity.

Keywords Metaphoricity • Metonymy • Structures of Feeling • Objet a • Desire • Pantemporality • Death Drive • Political Affect • Palimpsest • Intergenerational Transmission

> *When I come to shape here at this table between my hands the story of my life and set it before you as a complete thing, I have to recall things gone far, gone deep, sunk into this life or that and become part of it; dreams, too, things surrounding me, and the inmates, those old half-articulate ghosts who keep up their hauntings by day and night…shadows of people one might have been; unborn selves.*
> —Virginia Woolf

In his seminal work, *Marxism and Literature*, Raymond Williams describes "structures of feeling" as "social experiences in solution."[1] In contradistinction to "precipitated" affective experiences and semantic formations that are immediately available to conscious interpretation, the so-called structures of feeling exert a true influence on a society's general modalities of action and affective experience while sitting "at the very edge of seman-tic availability,"[2] appearing as articulations only occasionally. Even without delving into Williams' discussion of these spectral "structures," it is easy to notice intriguing connections between the idea of structures of feeling and such notions as hauntology as detailed by Derrida or the crypt and cryp-tonymy as developed by Abraham and Torok[3] in addressing intergenera-tional transmission of affective experiences. Lurking at the very edge of conscious availability, the ghost appears occasionally to represent another time and another place, and, when it haunts, even when it fully occupies the ego, it is perceived as imposing its structure on the here and now of subjective experience from the outside of the now and the here. While the double for instance can be seen as the figuration of individual, internal and intra-psychic processes,[4] the ghost is the manifestation of an affectively charged figuration borne of the collective, external and inter-psychic pro-cesses and representing the structural configurations of another time and hence another place—a fact that further highlights their relevance to the notion of structures of feeling.

systems as linguistic systems abstracted from the living experience of the subject—and to develop our theories and our analyses of experience and subjectivity accordingly. We need, in other words, to understand and incorporate into our formulation of subjective experience the fact that meaning as such is always-already haunted, and that we need to reformulate the two main outcomes of semiosis, namely temporality and desire, accordingly.

DESIRE, MEANING, AND TIME

The following quotation from the Austrian theologian, Friedrich von Hügel,[13] which Victor Turner once used to conclude a lecture on what he called "images of anti-temporality" would serve us as an apt point of entry into this question. Von Hügel wrote:

> Eternal Life, in the fullest thinkable sense, involves three things –the plentitude of all goods and of all energizings that abide; the entire self-consciousness of the Being Which constitutes and Which is expressed by all these goods and energizings; and the pure activity, the non-successiveness, the simultaneity, of this Being in all It has, all It is. Eternal Life, in this sense, precludes not only space, not only clock time- that artificial chain of mutually exclusive, ever equal moments, but even duration, time as actually experienced by man, with its overlapping, interpenetrating successive stages ... The Simultaneity is here the fullest expression of ... the unspeakable Concreteness ... and is at the opposite pole from all empty unity ... any or all abstractions whatsoever.[14]

I don't intend to address the topics of temporality and atemporality from a metaphysical point of view, nor even a philosophical one for that matter. Indeed one point that I would hope to at least implicitly drive home is the need for freeing the notion of atemporality from those exotic domains and bringing it into the very heart of the daily experience of human life, where social, political, ethnographic, and clinical inquiries typically look for their material. To put this in other words, rather than addressing such questions as the nature of time, whether it is continuous or discrete, or whether it is real or illusory, I addresses what Hegel termed "human time" or "historical time." What I am interested in addressing is the question of temporality and atemporality as experienced by the human mind, and the implications of that modality of experience for research and analysis, and more importantly for this book, its relevance to the notion of hauntology as an "everyday" process.

The excerpt Turner chose to quote from von Hügel addresses two notions that are fundamental in a discussion of human temporality. The first is what he terms "unspeakable concreteness," and the second, standing in opposition to the first, he describes as "any abstraction whatsoever." The evolutionary graph I discussed earlier and the trajectory of abstraction vs. concreteness aside, anyone familiar with the Lacanian school of psychoanalysis would be well aware of the significance these same two concepts hold in Lacan's thought, albeit articulated under the rubrics of "the real" and "the symbolic." Once juxtaposed with that frame of reference (a juxtaposition that does not require a real stretch of either idea, and thus elaboration here), we can simply read von Hügel to be stating that time is a product of symbolization, or in any case that time exists only within the order of the symbolic.[15]

The idea that temporality is a product of symbolization and meaning-making is both the basic point of departure for my discussion and a guiding principle. Before entering the discussion, however, it may be useful to set up another basic point of reference through another highly abbreviated account of the originary trajectory of the human subject from a Lacanian object relational point of view.[16]

Briefly (and again, not unrelated to the evolutionary graph I mentioned in the earlier chapter), the so-called trajectory can be thought to start with the serene, relatively static, and unconscious state of existence of the fetus growing as a purely physical/biological extension of the body of the mother, followed by a course of development culminating in a fundamental and violent separation from the mother's body initiated through a traumatic passage into the harsh and dynamic external world of sensations, images, objects, and eventually ideas, and of course symbols, language, subjects, and power. As humans we therefore start our individual journey from materiality to subjectivity with a package deal built around a profound separation/loss, a traumatic initiation, and an urgent need to develop novel capacities and behaviors such as breathing air, ingesting food, perceiving and recognizing "external" images and objects, and making noises and gestures to represent and to communicate our inner experiences, in order to survive through various levels of interaction with the material and the symbolic environments.

The "internal" force of biological survival appears to command and unfold its ways (from breathing air, ingestion of food and expulsion of feces, to crying and the range of pre-symbolic interactions) almost regardless of what else may be taking place in the environment. Yet that same internal force eventually conjoins the pre-existing external forces of the social realm (expressed through language and other symbolic structures), and together these two forces lead the human infant to submit to and to "internalize" cognitive and behavioral systems of meaningful action and communication—that is to say, to becoming a human social subject.

We can identify in this process of initiation of the infant within the realm of meaning and social self-consciousness two tendencies in different directions. The two tendencies are associated with and oriented on the one hand by a fundamental "separation" (think of both the literal trajectory of organic unity and eventual separation from mother's body, and the process of transformation of bodily sensation to symbolic and mental representations discussed in the last chapter) and the loss and "lack" which is created in its wake of and, and on the other hand by our species' evolved capacity to transform/replace that absence into the experience of a lost "object" (remember *das Ding*) and re-creating (representing) that "imagined" lost object within a realm of abstractions, the realm of symbolic reality, or meaning. Due to their seemingly differing orientations,[17] these two forces push or pull in different directions: one continuously "urges" or "pushes" the subject to venture further and further into the symbolic realm, or, in von Hügel's language, to the realm of "empty unity and abstraction," while the other constantly "harks" or "pulls" the subject back toward an imaginary silent "home" of unmediated presence—what von Hügel termed "unspeakable concreteness." These two forces are two basic elements that need to be deeply understood and theorized in developing a sense for the role of temporality in human experience, and in outlining a hauntological theory of subjective experience. Let's take a closer look.

The first force, born out of loss and manifested in the dynamics of abstraction and symbolization, is the force that drives the subject ceaselessly forward "in time," chasing after the ever elusive goal of reaching or reuniting with the lost object (arriving at satisfaction in various aspects of life, or arriving at a final and complete meaning in understanding of the self or the world). The missing "thing" is not an "actual" lost object of course, insofar as the so-called lost object itself is a product of the appearance of imagination and symbolization—again, think both the organic development of the infant's ego, and the semiotic emergence/expression of meaning and language. In both cases, the "Thing" in question is an always-already abstracted and represented lost object which is continuously reproduced through the projection of our lack of and hence our desire for it onto the world, in the fashion of a mirage—a mirage that, like any mirage, will never actually stand still and wait for us to reach it, because it does not really "exist," and so it can never be captured. I will return to this notion in more detail later (see Chap. 4) in discussing *objet a*. This is the process that Lacan is speaking about when he writes, "symbol manifests itself first of all as the killing of the thing, and this death results in the endless perpetuation of the subject's desire,"[18] or to go further back to the original idea, this is what Hegel means when he suggests, "all conceptual understanding is equivalent to a murder."[19]

Note that what I have just described includes a number of references to movement. Movement is a significant aspect of this force, in at least two respects: in the linguistic sense of the slippage of meaning, and in the psychoanalytic sense of the deference of desire. This is one field of subjective experience in which the private/psychological and the collective/linguistic coincide, specifically in terms of the continuous push of desire and the "movement" of meaning. The movement of meaning, or the "slippage of the signified" as Lacan put it,[20] is the incessant escape of the desired meaning through chains of metonymic association, and our continuous mental movement after the eternally deferred Meaning and its promise of the Truth. The psychological expression of this effect we term desire, and the linguistic effect is best captured under the rubric of metonymy. This also appears to be where the human experience of temporality is born. As a matter of fact, Alexandre Kojève's reading of Hegel[21] offers a very clear and useful interpretation of the interconnectedness of desire, symbolic projection, and time, which merits quoting in some detail before moving on to the linguistic interpretation of this account in terms of the logic of metonymy. Hegel, says Kojève,[22] argues that human subject's time (which, as mentioned earlier, he calls historic time, as opposed to biological or cosmic time) is characterized by the primacy of the future in its construction. He writes:

> In the Time that pre-Hegelian Philosophy considered, the movement went from the Past toward the Future, by way of the Present. In the Time of which Hegel speaks, on the other hand, the movement is engendered in the Future and goes toward the Present by way of the Past. And this is indeed the specific structure of properly human —that is, historical—Time. In fact, let us consider the phenomenological (or better, anthropological) projection

of this metaphysical analysis of Time. The movement engendered by the Future is the movement that arises from Desire. This means: from specifically human Desire –that is, creative Desire—that is, Desire that is directed toward an entity that does not exist and has not existed in the real natural World. Only then can the movement be said to be engendered by the Future, for the Future is precisely what does not (yet) exist and has not (already) existed... As a matter of fact, Desire is the presence of an absence: I am thirsty because there is an absence of water in me. It is indeed, then, the presence of a future in the present: of the future act of drinking....The being that acts thus, therefore, is in a Time in which the Future takes primacy. And inversely, the Future can really take primacy only if, in the real (spatial) world, there is a being capable of acting thus....Now, if Desire is the presence of an absence, it is not –taken as such—an empirical reality: it does not exist in a positive manner in the natural – i.e., spatial—Present. On the contrary, it is like a gap or a "hole" in Space: an emptiness, a nothingness.... Desire that is related to Desire, therefore, is related to nothing. To "realize" it, therefore, is to realize nothing. In being related only to the Future, one does not come to a reality, and consequently one is not really in motion... therefore, in order to realize itself, Desire must be related to a reality; but it cannot be related to it in a positive manner. Hence it must be related to it negatively. Therefore Desire is necessarily the Desire to negate the real or present given. And the reality of Desire comes from the negation of the given reality. Now, the negated real is the real that has ceased to be: it is the past real, or the real Past...Therefore, generally speaking: the historical movement arises from the Future and passes through the Past in order to realize itself in the Present or as temporal Present. The Time that Hegel has in view, then, is human or historical Time: it is the Time of conscious and voluntary action which realizes in the present a Project of the future, which Project is formed on the basis of knowledge of the past.[23]

What is detailed by Kojève here lies at the core of Lacan's semiotic conceptualization of desire—and of temporality. It includes the role of metonymic force in the dynamics of lack and the projection of the desired within the symbolic realm through the function of metonymy, but also the role of the metaphoric function, though it is not explicitly detailed here. "Metonymic structure," says Lacan, indicates "the signifier-to-signifier connection that allows for the elision by which the signifier instates lack of being [*le manque de l'être*] in the object-relation, using signification's referral [*renvoi*] value to invest it with the desire aiming at the lack that it supports."[24] With Lacan, Hegel, and Derrida, here we are at the center of where it all happens. It is this close understanding of the formation of desire and the role of the "lost" object which allows an appreciation of the true sense of hauntology as a descriptive formulation of meaning, time, and subjective experience as such—a hauntology that is relevant not just to grand events and traumatized minds, but to the everyday human experience of time and meaning.

THE METONYMIC FUNCTION

The basic idea of movement as an aspect of symbolization and expressed through the metonymic function directly associates the metonymic function with time and temporality, in multiple respects. Temporality of subjective experience is born out of the symbolization process not only in terms of the production/projection of the future and thus the establishment of the "future-past-present" cycle (which is of course experienced as a linear past-present-future by the subject), but also in terms of the introduction of a sense of a lost object in the past tense on the one hand, and the repeated deferral into future of meaning across the chain of signifiers on the other; as well as both the physical and syntactical expressions of the metonymic function, namely that it is only through the unfolding in time of meaning along sets and units of signification, such as a sentence, a word, or even a phoneme, that meaning is communicated. Signification proceeds in a linear timeline before its meaning is complete,[25] a temporality that "seem[s] oddly smooth and characterless – 'pure' displacement, 'pure' continuity, a slippage or a passage that moves ahead with unstoppable fluency."[26] Meaning and the communication of it are possible only in time, and this is what Lacan means when he says, "the name is the time of the object."[27] The name, or the word, to go back to Hegel, kills the object, but gives it time and sets the stage for its return through the haunted meaning. Of interest in this formulation of desire, meaning, object and subject is also an idea not examined by Kojève, but later picked up by Lacan, namely *objet a*. Closely tied to *das Ding* in its formation and function, *objet a* can be understood as a projected object of desire which is unreal insofar as it is a creation of fantasy, and yet real enough insofar as it functions both as desire's point of reference (or its cause, as Lacan likes to put it) in future, and as the pivot around which meaning is anchored. *Objet a*'s unique ontology (its hauntology, to be precise) lends itself directly to a powerful formulation of ghosts and the phenomenon of haunting as caused by abrupt disruptions of *objet a*, which I will address in the next chapter.

To recap the basic points of interest here then, a projective force is recognizable in the metonymic function of the order of signification, and the ever-lasting slippage away of the object cause of desire through an endless deferral of meaning on the axis of metonymy. This is precisely what Lacan means when he asserts boldly that "desire is a metonymy."[28] This is also the ultimate "deception" of the symbolic order, whose endless labyrinth we naively and eagerly spend our lives searching for the lost "beloved," to borrow from poetic and religious terminology—the beloved that never was, indeed whose very existence has become possible through our capacity to produce and to engage the so-called labyrinth. This is the force that has pushed us forward to create more and more complicated mazes of ideas and concepts, to philosophize, to think up more lofty and more intricate logical edifices, with the insatiable hope/desire of someday somehow arriving at the lost object of our imagination, typically personified in utopian terms such as paradise, love, happiness, justice, freedom, the classless society, the pure society, et cetera.

THE METAPHORIC FUNCTION

Let us consider now what I described earlier as a second force. This force functions and pulls in what appears as a radically different direction, by the fascinating effect of "cutting" or "jumping" through the layers of signification, and offering the promise of thus connecting us in an immediate fashion to that which we have lost, and which we somehow experience as belonging in "the past" and located in "the deep." This second function is different from the metonymic function in that, rather than urging to go further and to construct more complex layers of abstraction in search of that which we have supposedly lost, it harks *back* to a mysterious place associated more with depth than height, more with darkness than light, with past than future, with nostalgia than anticipation, and, to go back again to von Hügel, with the concrete than with the abstract. This second force can be recognized at work in what Lacan identifies as the metaphoric function, which differs from the metonymic function primarily in terms of its relationship to the real: "no one," insists Lacan, "has yet validly articulated what links metaphor to the question of being, and metonymy to its lack."[29] The very fact that such a question should arise, however, is sufficiently telling for the purposes of our discussion, namely the divergent "directions" of the two forces: whereas metonymy unfolds in time and constitutes the death of the object, metaphor offers to somehow "link back" to the lost object, and promises the timeless. Little wonder that metaphor so often serves across literary genres as a favorite gateway for ghosts to return and haunt—literally or metaphorically.

Metaphor, believes Lacan, functions like a "spark," leaping across two signifiers that are not otherwise associated, and in so doing it cuts across the linear relations that govern the metonymic system. But more importantly, metaphor also breaks through the "bar" that separates the signifier from the signified, the subject from its experience.[30] What is most relevantly significant about this aspect of metaphor is that in its performance it breaches the boundaries of the purely symbolic register and reaches through the so-called imaginary order toward von Hügel's total concreteness, or the real, as Lacan would name it. You may recall from the last chapter that this resonates clearly with the more basic function served by phonemes as they bridge the bodily order to the linguistic order to make possible the linguistic function as such. Metaphors seem to perform a similar bridging task, albeit at a higher level of organization. Like the phonemic function which serves as both constituent and a gateway for the "ghost" of the thing to haunt meaning, the metaphoric function serves as both constituent and a gateway for the ghost of the lost object (of imagination and desire) to haunt the subject's thought and experience.

Ricoeur, even though looking at metaphors from a substantially different angle, describes them in terms directly relevant to and resonant with this formulation. "Thanks to its character as half thought and half experience," he writes in *The Role of Metaphor*, "metaphor joins the light of sense with the fullness of the image." And he goes on to add, "in this way, the non-verbal and the verbal are firmly united at the core of the imaging function of language."[31] What Ricoeur addresses in this formulation is a fundamental aspect of metaphor that makes possible its role in a process through which meaning is completed—the same process through which the quality of pantemporality is introduced into the otherwise linear temporality of the metonymic function. That fundamental aspect is due to the amphibian or liminal nature of metaphor: it simultaneously belongs to the symbolic and the imaginary orders of perception. In fact Ricoeur later dedicated a full article to expanding on this basic quality of the metaphoric process.[32] He insists that the nature of metaphor constitutes a case against the "well-established dichotomy" between "sense" as the objective content of an expression and "representation" as the "mental actualization ... in the form of image and feeling."[33]

THANATOS AND EROS

Before examining the relevance of metonymic and metaphoric functions to the question of pantemporality in more detail, another feature of this dichotomy merits mention, namely its apparent coincidence with Freud's famous yet less understood binary, Thanatos and Eros. A detailed comparative examination would fall beyond the interest of my discussion, but the way in which the two binary pairs can be readily tied to each other is sufficiently significant (and evident) to be addressed in passing. Here is how Freud originally introduced the idea:

> On the basis of theoretical considerations, supported by biology, we put forward the hypothesis of a death instinct, the task of which is to lead organic life back into the inanimate state; on the other hand, we supposed that Eros, by bringing about a more and more far-reaching combination of the particles into which living substance is dispersed, aims at complicating life and at the same time, of course, at preserving it.[34]

At the first glance this passage appears to coincide quite seamlessly with the two forces I have described in terms of the metonymic and metaphoric functions: the metaphoric function seems to coincide with Thanatos or the "death instinct," pulling as it does toward an origin of concrete, lifeless serenity; while the metonymic function sounds like another way of describing Eros, the "life instinct" continuously producing "more and more far-reaching combination of the particles." In fact elsewhere Freud speaks still more specifically of this binary opposition between a force that pushes toward complexity and abstraction, and one that pushes toward a return to the original state of concrete substance (and let's not ignore the strong resonance here with Von Uexküll). Freud writes:

> The attributes of life were at some time evoked in inanimate matter by the action of a force of whose nature we can form no conception. It may perhaps have been a process similar in type to that which later caused the development of consciousness in a particular stratum of living matter. The tension which then arose in what had hitherto been an inanimate substance endeavored to cancel itself out. In this way the first instinct came into being: the instinct to return to the inanimate state.[35]

We would be well advised of course to avoid rash leaps here. It is important, for instance, to recall that both the metaphoric and the metonymic functions come to exist and function within the realm of the symbolic (the "Janusian" function of metaphor notwithstanding), while Eros and Thanatos have to be conceptualized as primal processes far predating the appearance of the (human) symbolic order. Given the clear parallelism between the structural functions and directions of the two forces, however, it does appear safe to hypothesize the metaphoric and metonymic forces as counterparts to Thanatos and Eros respectively, within the register of abstractions. In other words, while the metonymic force may be understood as the expression of the negative (see Kojève above) through the function of Eros, the metaphoric force can be thought of as the expression of the negative through the function of Thanatos. If such formulation appears too paradoxical to hold, it might be helpful to recall Freud's own assertion that "the aim of all life is death"[36] and compare that with the earlier description here, that both the metaphoric and the metonymic forces are indeed aiming at a return to the "original" state. The paradox, it seems, is integral to the process in a fundamental way.

Elsewhere, in *Civilization and its Discontents*, Freud sets the basic force that causes the development of the ego and leads to the creation of law, order, and civilization as such, against a second force that draws some to "a sensation of eternity, a feeling as of something limitless, unbounded, something oceanic."[37] In fact Freud uses the coexistence of the two tendencies and the two modalities of experience to outline a pantemporal[38] psychic apparatus in which "the original type of feeling survives alongside the later one."[39] He goes into some length to argue for the existence of such pantemporality by drawing analogies from the simultaneous presence of qualities belonging to various stages of evolution/history in the same species or the same place. He uses the powerful imagery of "the Timeless City" to drive the point home: "the fantastic supposition that Rome were not a human dwelling-place, but a mental entity with just as long and varied a past history: that is, in which nothing once constructed had perished, and all the earlier stages of development had survived alongside the latest."[40]

The "creative spark" of metaphor, elaborates Lacan, is not created by the simple juxtaposition of two images or two signifiers. The spark flashes, he says, "between two signifiers, one of which has replaced the other by taking the other's place in the signifying chain, the occulted signifier remaining present by virtue of its (metonymic) connection to the rest of the chain."[41] Consider the idea that an "occulted signifier" remains "present" through the new signifier, and the implications of this in terms of temporality, in the sense that something of the supposedly bygone past remains present outside of the expected flow of time—leaving us little choice but to think about ghosts and haunting.

THE HAUNTED METAPHOR

In a separate remark paralleling the assertion I mentioned earlier, that "desire is a metonymy," Lacan also asserts "the symptom is a metaphor"[42] or elsewhere, "metaphor [is] but a synonym for the symbolic displacement brought into play in the symptom."[43] Compacted in these statements is a formulation that connects metaphor directly to repressed concepts, experiences and memories, and more generally to ghosts, to times out of joint, and a past that is present. As indicated earlier in passing, the idea of present pasts had been expressed powerfully by Freud on numerous occasions where he insisted on the pantemporality (atemporality, to use his own words) of the psychic apparatus. He writes in *Civilization and Its Discontents*:

> Since the time when we recognized the error of supposing that ordinary forgetting signified destruction or annihilation of the memory-trace, we have been inclined to the opposite view that nothing once formed in the mind could ever perish, that everything survives in some way or other, and is capable under certain conditions of being brought to light again, as, for instance, when regression extends back far enough.[44]

What Lacan's work has made possible for us, however, is a closer and clearer formulation of the mechanics of this pantemporality, specifically in linguistic and semiotic terms, and specifically through the intersections of the metaphoric and metonymic functions. To go back to Ricoeur, the major function of metaphor is creating a shortcut in the temporal/spatial distance between two terms:

> It is as though a change of distance between meanings occurred within a logical space. The new pertinence or congruence proper to a meaningful metaphoric utterance proceeds from the kind of semantic proximity which suddenly obtains between terms in spite of their distance. Things or ideas which were remote appear now as close . . . [a] move or shift in the logical distance, from the far to the near.[45]

Insofar as the psychological functions are concerned then, specifically insofar as "feelings" are directly associated with and connected to these semiotic "terms" that metaphor magically ties to one another, the metaphoric function constitutes a semi-permeable passage through which "the past" is able to invade or possess the present at any given time. This is precisely what makes the psychoanalytic function of transference, this most basic function observable in the clinical setting, possible. On the other hand, what constantly resists and stops such invasion of the past from a full takeover of the present is the force of the syntactic cohesion of language/thought held together through "chains" of signification. The primary force of binding that links the terms of these so-called chains together is provided through the metonymic function, which constantly "struggles" to avoid, to cover, and to deny the existence of the real as that which calls from the past and the depth of language through the imaginary. Ironically, of course, the metonymic function alone is not capable of holding the system of thought and meaning together in the live sense that is experienced by the subject, it is only with the intervention of the metaphoric function that the ensemble of language as a combination of *la langue* and *parole*[46] is mobilized, specifically around *objet a* and through the anchoring function of *points de capiton*.[47] To recap then, metonymy functions on the horizontal axis,[48] works/unfolds through time, sustains the experience of linear temporality, and perpetuates the work/flow of desire in a never ending deferral of sense; while metaphor functions on the vertical axis, cuts/jumps through experienced temporality, is closely associated with the psychic functions of condensation, repression, and transference, and acts as a time tunnel or a palimpsest always-already "symptomatic," always-already haunted.

It would be useful to reiterate here the basic feature of metaphor that is central to this discussion, namely that metaphors are simultaneously linguistic tropes and seats of experience. Metaphor, according to Ricoeur, achieves a modality of "fusion" between "sense [meaning] and sensa [sense data]"[49] or of "sense and the imaginary"[50] or, as he elaborates elsewhere, of "thinking and feeling."[51] To translate Ricoeur's idea into the Lacanian triadic model, we can say metaphor has two faces, one of which appears in the realm of the imaginary, the other in the realm of the symbolic. This is exactly why and how for Lacan "symptom is a metaphor," in the sense that it is not simply a representation of a psychic fact or past experience, it is simultaneously a representation (of the past) and an experience (in presence). Or to go back to Victor Turner's work, this is the feature that allows the "anti-temporal stretch" of liminality to function as metaphor, to connect the two realms of the temporal and ordered (the symbolic) and the atemporal and not ordered according to the norms (imaginary), and also to invest signifiers with "other" meanings.[52] Let us remember here also that for Lacan one of metaphor's major functions is condensation: "what Freud calls condensation is what in rhetoric one calls metaphor."[53] Calling to mind Freud's work on the pantemporality of condensation (as in his discussion of the Timeless City, etc.), we seem to have arrived at a model capable of detailing the mechanics by which the quality of pantemporality becomes possible in an otherwise linear process of signification and subjective experience, and along with it, the inescapably haunted nature of meaning and subjective experience. We are, in other words, at the point of making better sense of Virginia Woolf's lamentation:

> When I come to shape here at this table between my hands the story of my life and set it before you as a complete thing, I have to recall things gone far, gone deep, sunk into this life or that and become part of it; dreams, too, things surrounding me, and the inmates, those old half-articulate ghosts who keep up their hauntings by day and night...shadows of people one might have been; unborn selves.[54]

Walter Benjamin says in one of his typically powerful observations, "allegories are, in the realm of thoughts, what ruins are in the realm of things."[55] Let us not miss the point that allegory is a supreme form of metaphor. Allegory, says Craig Owen, is "defined as a single metaphor introduced in continuous series."[56] And let us also keep in mind that allegory literally means "the other speaking."[57] It is, in other words, the repressed voice of an "other" signifier that haunts the signifier to turn it into a metaphor. Allegory, that elongated metaphor, says Owens, is "an attitude as well as a technique," "a perception as well as a procedure."[58] This is the function that renders metaphoricity an important point of interest in research, treatment and analysis of subjective experience as fundamentally haunted.

POLITICAL AFFECT

Due to its linguistic nature, metaphor also serves the important purpose of anchoring the subjective experience within the collective frame of reference. Lest we should forget, a "competition" between the metonymic and the metaphoric forces, said Jakobson "is manifest in any symbolic process, be it intrapersonal or social."[59] No less significantly, however, due to its unique temporal disposition as a palimpsest, metaphor also holds the subject and subjective experience afloat in a pantemporal universe where all past is always present. One feature of metaphor that becomes clear from these facts is that the past that inhabits metaphor is not simply the personal past or the past of speech (*parole*), but also the collective past, the past of language (*la langue*). This significant feature takes us back to the discussions with which this chapter opened, namely the hauntological natures of political affect and intergenerational transmission of affect.

In his book, *Political Affect: Connecting the Social and the Somatic*, John Protevi proposes to develop a way to think of human subjects as simultaneously collective and emotional but also individual and rational, by using the notions of "political physiology" and "political affect."[60] The notion of political physiology, he explains, submerges the field of "affective neuroscience" into a political context that recognizes "emergent social groups" and other "heterogeneous assemblages" above and alongside the subject.[61] Building strongly on the texts and theoretic models of Gilles Deleuze, Protevi suggests politics intersects with psychology and physiology via a "socially embedded and somatically embodied affective cognition."[62] The somatic, in other words, plays a central role in Protevi's understanding of the political and the affective. The affective is somatically based, and the political reaches and shapes the affective not through the symbolic system, but through the structuration of the somatic (hence the foundational place of "political physiology"). Even though in first glance Protevi's work seems to resonate closely and lend direct support to the notions of political subjectivity and political affect as formulated here, a closer look will show some conflicting premises, which may be helpful to clarifying my point here. One of the ways in which Protevi's approach contradicts what I am outlining here is explicitly stated in *Political Affect*. After describing his stance as one based on the "neomaterialist standpoint of Deleuze," he emphasizes that such a standpoint requires "that we turn away from a postphenomenological stance in which the real is only a retrojected effect of entering signifying systems."[63] While Protevi's reference in this passage is most likely to the line of work and ideas associated with Don Ihde's postphenomenology and techno-bodies,[64] it collides also with the underlying premises here, specifically those formulated within a Lacanian model of the relationship between the real, the imaginary, and the symbolic registers. The contrast becomes sharp around the role of the symbolic order and various semiotic mechanisms in formation of experience and subjectivity, and hence the formulation of the ways in which temporality, power, and the political find their ways into the subjective and the experiential, specifically within the framework of hauntology.

Protevi's work is by far too intricate to be briefly reacted to here, and too sophisticated to be simply set up in contrast to an aspect of my discussions here, but I have nonetheless decided to address it because it provides an important point of reference for anyone interested in this rapidly evolving conversation on subjectivity and political affect. Whereas in the context of my work[65] subjectivity is the point of interest for studying the relationship between the political, the psychological, and the historical, Protevi clearly claims that when it comes to basic affect "the conscious subject is bypassed in favor of an immediate link between a social trigger and a somatic mechanism."[66] The political, in this model, influences subjectivity not through higher level symbolic (semiotic, linguistic, etc.) mechanisms, but by directly impacting the body and "triggering" affects through its somatic impact. As I have discussed in the last chapter, the somatic undoubtedly continues to exert an influence within the symbolic realm, but the key difference would be that its influence is exerted through forces of spectrality, and via the hauntological nature of meaning, as we have seen for instance in examining phonemes and metaphors. The attribution of a direct interaction between the somatic and the political, however, is what Protevi calls "my claim to originality," and describes in terms of grounding individual rights and common good in "affective cognition as the sense-making of bodies politic rather than in a rational cognitive subject as the political subject."[67]

In short, while the notion of political affect as developed by Protevi clearly recognizes the formative role of structures of power in the work of affect, the idea of political affect as outlined here remains distinct from Protevi's, at least insofar as the nature and mechanisms of its politicality are concerned. Having said that, it is worth mentioning that some recent lines of work, such as Lisa Blackman's intriguing notion of "immaterial body"[68] seem to go a long way in addressing precisely the gaps between these two modalities—keep in mind the emphasis placed here on the role

ınd its nature, as it ties the somatic to the symbolic via the
ınphasis that may connect the two models in more ways
eye.
..un of affect as used here could perhaps be understood most
..urately in terms employed by Raymond Williams, as he formulated his
notion of "structures of feeling" as a collectively informed (infra)structure
that regulates our subjective modes of experience and modalities of par-
ticipation in social processes. Significantly, this approach would bypass the
discussion of what precisely constitutes affect, to address the mechanisms
involved in the formation of affect, and hence of subjective experience.
Structures of feeling in Williams view are "social experiences in solution,
as distinct from other social semantic formations which have been precipitated and are more evidently and more immediately available."[69] As the
discussion brings us back to the questions of hauntology and transmission
of affect, I would like also to make an undeservedly brief mention of the
work of Mark Fisher here, in which we can find the beginnings of an ideal
convergence of these themes of interest toward a more comprehensive
model for hauntology.

NETWORKED SUBJECTIVITY AND VIRTUAL AGENCY

In his brilliant treatment of what one might think of as a stoppage of rapid
change, and an abrupt end to the twentieth century's defining fantasy of
"progress," Mark Fisher traces a picture of the twenty-first century as a
haunted era, one in which a more or less finite set of structures of feeling
continue to be reproduced by each coming generation, as if haunted by a
history that has just fallen victim to its unanticipated end—to the cancel-
lation of its future. The reliance of contemporary artists on styles and
modalities that have been established long times ago, he says, is an indica-
tion of the fact that "the current moment is in the grip of a formal nostalgia."[70] Due to the fundamental changes in the very structure of our
subjective experience caused specifically by new technologies and post-
capitalist modes of production, culture has "lost its ability to grasp and
articulate the present," he believes.[71] I would suggest it is this very capacity of "grasping and articulating the present" that has always enabled culture to produce unique and temporally distinct sets of structures of affect,
which would serve in turn to produce the internal, subjective experience
of movement in time and the unfolding of history. It is also due to this
specific dysfunction of culture (as the source and holder of sign systems,

and hence as the "enactor" of our collective fantasies) that we are witnessing a breakdown of "the very distinction between past and present," and a social reality in which "cultural time has folded back on itself, and the impression of linear development has given way to a strange simultaneity."[72] And it is in terms of this formulation of the post-capitalist state of culture that hauntology offers the most appropriate conceptual tool in analysis of culture and subjectivity, even as the uncanny is no longer implied by the disjointment that is becoming the norm of our temporality. This hauntology may no longer be associated with (or at least limited to) the metaphysical and the supernatural, but nor is it simply a figure of speech: this hauntology is a means of addressing one of the foundational qualities of human subjectivity—a quality that has always lied at the core of what it is to be human, but is now, due to new technologies of information and new modalities of production, emerging as a defining feature of the twenty-first-century experience of *networked subjectivity.*

An effective approach to conceptualization of hauntology may be found in what Fisher calls "the agency of the virtual."[73] Such conceptualization has direct utility in analyzing technology's role in subjective experience, specifically toward the development of an analytic model for the emerging networked subjectivity, and perhaps beyond that, for conceptualization of artificial subjectivity. I consider both the emerging phenomenon of networked subjectivity and the theoretical conceptualization of artificial subjectivity important topics, to which I intend to dedicate more detailed attention in a future volume. More immediately, however, Fisher's notion of the agency of the virtual is also quite useful in conceptualization of ghosts as virtual agents of structures of feeling whose agency is effectuated not through biological/concrete existence, but through the virtual work of culture and fantasy, specifically the work of language and the symbolic system through such functions as metaphoricity, desire and *objet a*; but also through newly available modes of virtuality due to technologies of information, communication, and perception. It is also in precisely this sense that we recognize the close ties of the notion of intergenerational transmission of trauma with hauntology, structures of affect, and subjective experience. Both Freud and Marx, claimed Fisher, "had discovered different modes of this spectral causality."[74] Recalling the two forces suggested earlier, one may say that while Marx built his future-oriented theory on the ghosts of things to come (as in the specter of communism, anticipation of the effects of abstracted capital, and so on), Freud's hauntological edifice concerned itself with the past: (un)dead memories and moments, and the effect held on the present of the subject by ghosts of the object lost to the past. With the deep entrenchment of the postmodern condition in contemporary experiences of human subjectivity, it is no longer simply through the mechanisms identified by Marx and Freud, but more substantially through new technologies of virtuality and post-capitalist modes of production, meaning, and consumption that the question of hauntology gains new significance. Put in other words, it is as the transmission of affect becomes the central (if circular and networked) mode of (re)production of political affect and (a)historical memory in what one might consider the event horizon of human history, that hauntology, or the need for a hauntological understanding, rises to great urgency unlike ever before. And it is in recognition of the emergence of new modalities of human temporality that the notion of pantemporality of experience moves to take the center point as a quality understanding which is the prerequisite to developing new ways of understanding the subject of contemporary human experience.

We have long faced accumulating evidence that the processes of inter-generational transmission of affect, specifically unprocessed affect associated with collective experiences of strife and trauma (war, genocide, slavery, colonialism, etc.), greatly contribute to psychological, social, and political experiences at both group and individual levels. The lines of work spearheaded by Byron J. Good in cultural and psychological anthropology,[75] or those by Valerie Walkerdine and Lisa Blackman in social psychology, body, and media studies[76] offer brilliant examples of such evidence. In parallel with—and as a result of—that advancement, however, we have also been facing the growing awareness that we do not have either theoretical or methodological approaches capable of accounting for the day-to-day process of intergenerational transmission of affective and subjective patterns; and that what we do have, such as cognitive and behavioral or even traditional psychoanalytic models, are simply not effective or specific enough to give us clear methodological and analytic roadmaps. In fact basic technological and historical developments seem to have brought us to a point that leaves no option but to take seriously the hauntological nature of human subjectivity at large, and "the agency of the virtual," or at any rate, the incessant work of virtual agents in patterning our psychological processes and our political affect. We are at a point where we can no longer ignore the need for theories and models that would enable us to understand "the specificity of material and discursive conditions under which lives are led," as Walkerdine puts it, "the practices and embodied and affective responses that ensue, the ways that those embodiments are passed down generations, and the practices, tropes, and fantasies that both sustain and break apart communities and families."[77] We are, in other words, in need of a hauntological theory of the everyday life.

Insofar as the semiotic and symbolic underpinnings of the processes addressed here constitute the foundational mechanisms of subjectivity, this model has two basic corollaries: (1) it seamlessly connects individual experience not simply to the personal past but also to the collective past, and (2) it brings the theory of that relationship down to the level of everyday life. Even without delving deeply into these two important implications, it is easy enough to see the direct relevance of this model to the study and analysis of topics ranging from political subjectivity and intergenerational transmission of (political) affect to issues of collective trauma, ghosts and haunting, political group processes and impact of history on current affairs, and more. These topics have traditionally been thought of as "analyzable" in association with outstanding and excessive events of history—again, in both the clinical sense of personal history and the anthropological sense of collective history, such as great loss and mourning, personal trauma, as well as colonialism, natural disasters, wars, genocides or what Michael M.J. Fischer has called "post-trauma societies."[78] A hauntological understanding of the linguistic/semiotic underpinnings of pantemporality as outlined here, however, makes it clear that the process is by far more ordinary and abundant than are such grand events, insofar as it is the very basic condition for the appearance and functioning of meaning, time, and subjective experience. As indicated in passing here and also hinted at by Mark Fisher's reference to "spectral causality" in Freud,[79] it is possible for instance to argue for an identification of the metaphoric function almost directly with the process of transference, the foundational modality of subjective experience in psychoanalytic work. The "magic" that makes possible the function of transference is precisely the same magic that makes possible the function of metaphor. After all, in both processes one object, one signifier, is possessed by another and is understood in terms of the other. "What are transferences?" asked Freud in *Fragment of an Analysis of a Case of Hysteria*, and he then answered himself:

[Transferences] are new editions or facsimiles of the impulses and fantasies .... but they have this peculiarity which is characteristic for their species, that they replace some earlier person by the person of the physician. To put it another way: a whole series of psychological experiences are revived, not as belonging to the past, but as applying to the person of the physician at the present moment. Some of these transferences have a content which differs from that of their model in no respect whatever except for substitution. These then –to keep to the same metaphor—are merely new impressions or reprints.[80]

In his later work and through abundant experience Freud realizes the predominance of the mechanism of transference as a foundational aspect of everyday cognition and subjective experience as such. In *An Autobiographical Study*, for instance, he speaks of transference as a "universal phenomenon of the human mind" that "dominates the whole of each person's relations to his human environment."[81]

The scope and reach of the notion of pantemporality as the phenomenological stage on which hauntology emerges are simply too far reaching to exhaust here. For that same reason, however, it is also imperative that we arrive at a robust understanding of the processes involved, that we theorize them extensively, and that we introduce them into our analytic methodology at a foundational level. If this chapter has made one point only, I would want that to be the need for releasing our conceptualization of temporality in subjective experience from the reductive synchronic-vs.-diachronic binarism, and to consider the abundant evidence that pantemporality is a fundamental feature of human experience of meaning and subjectivity. The need has become similarly inevitable, I hope, for a model of subjectivity that liberates the subject from the binds of individual vs. collective dualism and recognizes the subject as that which is the interface of the two. In light of this reading, such enigmas as ghosts, haunting, and present pasts can finally be rightly understood to be not just about exotic places, exotic histories, excessive events, or severe psychological states, but about here and now, about me and about you, and present at the most basic levels of culture and history. The time, we need to learn to appreciate, is always out of joint in some sense, and everything that we have to say about the now would be grossly incomplete, until we locate and outline that now in the presence of its numerous pasts. As the past is accountable to the present, so the present is accountable to the past—through the future.

NOTES

1. Williams, 1977, p. 133.
2. Ibid.
3. See Abraham and Torok, 1994, 2005.
4. See Rahimi, 2013.
5. Williams, 1977, p. 128.
6. Williams, 1977.
7. Berthin, 2010, pp. 5–6.
8. Derrida, 2001a, p. 398.
9. Davis, 2007, p. 13.
10. Derrida, 2001b, p. 42.
11. Wolfreys, 2002, p. 3.
12. Blackman et al., 2008.
13. Friedrich von Hügel, aka Baron von Hügel (1852–1925), Austrian Roman Catholic theologian.
14. Quoted in Turner, 1982, pp. 264–5.
15. I would like to emphasize once more that this and all future references to "time" need to be read as "time as experienced by the human subject," and not the general concept of time as such.
16. I will refrain from discussing in great details or extensive referencing in the interest of brevity here, but interested readers can consult for instance Freud (1900), Jones (1948), Klein (1939, 1952, 1975), Bion (1962a, b), Lacan (1981a, 1996), or Kristeva (1989) for elaborations on these concepts.
17. Even though for all intents and purposes these are one and the same force, simply expressed in different directions. Think of the two sides of a single arch in a magnetic force field, which appear as if organized by two distinct forces flowing in different directions.
18. Lacan, 1953, p. 262.
19. Kojève 1969, p. 140.
20. Lacan, 1957, p. 419.
21. Kojève, 1969.
22. It may be worth mentioning that this segment of Kojève's course is supposedly his re-articulation of a reading of Hegel done by yet another Franco-Russian Hegelist, Alexandre Koyré.
23. Kojève 1969, pp. 134–6.
24. Lacan, 1957, p. 428.
25. Albeit not before the intervention of metaphor through what Lacan termed *points de capiton*. See below.
26. Bowie, 1991, p. 179.
27. Lacan, 1988, p. 169.

28. Lacan, 1957, p. 439.
29. Lacan, 1957, p. 439.
30. Lacan, 1957, p. 422.
31. Ricoeur, 1975, p. 253.
32. See Ricoeur (1978) The Metaphorical Process as Cognition, Imagination, and Feeling.
33. Ricoeur, 1978, p. 144.
34. Freud, 1923, p. 40.
35. Freud, 1920, p. 32.
36. Freud, 1920, p. 32.
37. See Freud, 1929, pp. 3ff.
38. Pantemporality is not Freud's terminology.
39. Freud, 1929, p. 3.
40. Freud, 1929, pp. 4–5.
41. Lacan, 1957, p. 422.
42. Lacan, 1957, p. 422.
43. Lacan, 1957, p. 216.
44. Freud, 1929, p. 4.
45. Ricoeur, 1978, p. 147.
46. Saussure, 1959.
47. See next chapter for further discussion.
48. The double-axes model referred to here is derived originally from the teachings of de Saussure and used then by both Jakobson and Lacan. The model consists of a horizontal axis, A-B, which Saussure termed the axis of simultaneities, and a vertical axis, C-D, which he termed the axis of successions (see Saussure, 1959, pp. 78ff). Whereas the axis of simultaneities "stands for the relations of coexisting things" (i.e. signifiers in a system of signs), on the axis of successions "only one thing can be considered at a time, but upon [it] are located all the things on the first axis together with their changes" (Ibid., p. 79). The setup and theorizing of these axes and their function have changed from Saussure to Jakobson to Lacan, and remain a point of occasional dispute. The discussion in this text is built around the Lacanian model.
49. Ricoeur, 1975, p. 250.
50. Ricoeur, 1975, p. 253.
51. Ricoeur, 1978, p. 147.
52. Turner, 1982, p. 250.
53. Lacan, 1981b, p. 252.
54. Woolf, 2005, p. 775.
55. Benjamin, 1998, p. 178.
56. Owens, 1980, p. 72.
57. From Greek: *allos* (other) + -*agoria* (speaking).

58. Owens, 1980, p. 68.
59. Jakobson, 1956, p. 258.
60. Protevi, 2009, p. 186.
61. Protevi, 2009, p. 188.
62. Protevi, 2009, p. vii.
63. Protevi, 2009, p. vii.
64. See e.g. Ihde 1995, 2002.
65. See for instance Rahimi, 2015a, b.
66. Protevi, 2009, p. 187.
67. Protevi, 2009, p. 185.
68. E.g. Blackman, 2012; Blackman and Venn, 2010.
69. Williams, 1977, pp. 133–134.
70. Fisher, 2014, p. 30.
71. Fisher, 2014, p. 31.
72. Fisher, 2014, p. 33.
73. Fisher, 2014, p. 47.
74. Fisher, 2014, p. 47.
75. See e.g. Good, 2015, 2019; Good and DelVecchio-Good, 2008.
76. See e.g. Walkerdine, 2015; Walkerdine et al., 2013; Blackman, 2012, 2019.
77. Walkerdine, 2015, p. 169.
78. Fischer, 1991.
79. Fisher, 2014, 47.
80. Freud, 1905, p. 116.
81. Freud, 1925, p. 42.

References

Abraham, N., & Torok, M. (1994). *The Shell and the Kernel: Renewals of Psychoanalysis* (Vol. 1). Trans. N. T. Rand. University of Chicago Press.

Abraham, N., & Torok, M. (2005). *The Wolf Man's Magic Word: A Cryptonymy.* University of Minnesota Press.

Benjamin, W. (1998). *The Origin of German Tragic Drama.* Verso.

Berthin, C. (2010). *Gothic Hauntings: Melancholy Crypts and Textual Ghosts.* Palgrave Macmillan.

Bion, W. R. (1962a). *Learning from Experience.* Tavistock.

Bion, W. R. (1962b). The psycho-analytic study of thinking. *International Journal of Psycho-Analysis, 43,* 306–310.

Blackman, L. (2012). *Immaterial Bodies: Affect, Embodiment, Mediation.* Sage.

Blackman, L. (2019). *Haunted Data: Affect, Transmedia, Weird Science.* Bloomsbury Publishing.

Blackman, L., & Venn, C. (2010). Affect. *Body and Society, 16*(1), 7–28.

Blackman, L., Cromby, J., Hook, D., Papadopulos, D., & Walkerdine, V. (2008). Creating Subjectivities. *Subjectivity, 22,* 1–27.

Bowie, M. (1991). *Lacan.* Harvard University Press.

Davis, C. (2007). *Haunted Subjects: Deconstruction, Psychoanalysis and the Return of the Dead.* Palgrave Macmillan.

Derrida, J. (2001a). *Papier Machine.* Galilée.

Derrida, J. (2001b). *The Work of Mourning.* University of Chicago Press.

Fischer, M. M. (1991). Anthropology as Cultural Critique: Inserts for the 1990s Cultural Studies of Science, Visual-Virtual Realities, and Post-Trauma Polities. *Cultural Anthropology, 6,* 525–537.

Fisher, M. (2014). *Ghosts of My Life: Writings on Depression, Hauntology and Lost Futures.* John Hunt Publishing.

Freud, S. (1900). The Interpretation of Dreams. In J. Strachey (Ed. & Trans.), *Standard Edition of the Complete Psychological Works of Sigmund Freud* (Vol. IV, pp. 1–338). Hogarth Press.

Freud, S. (1905). Fragment of an Analysis of a Case of Hysteria. In J. Strachey (Ed. & Trans.), *Standard Edition of the Complete Psychological Works of Sigmund Freud* (Vol. VII, pp. 7–122). Hogarth Press.

Freud, S. (1920). *Beyond the Pleasure Principle.* W.W. Norton and Company.

Freud, S. (1923). The Ego and the ID. In J. Strachey (Ed. & Trans.), *Standard Edition of the Complete Psychological Works of Sigmund Freud* (Vol. XIX, pp. 1–66). Hogarth Press.

Freud, S. (1925). An Autobiographical Study. In J. Strachey (Ed. & Trans.), *Standard Edition of the Complete Psychological Works of Sigmund Freud* (Vol. XX, pp. 7–74). Hogarth Press.

Freud, S. (1929). *Civilization and Its Discontents.* Chrysoma Associates.

Good, B. J. (2015). Haunted by Aceh: Specters of Violence in Post-Suharto Indonesia. In D. E. Hinton & A. L. Hinton (Eds.), *Genocide and Mass Violence: Memory, Symptom, and Recovery* (pp. 58–82). Cambridge University Press.

Good, B. J. (2019). Hauntology: Theorizing the Spectral in Psychological Anthropology. *Ethos, 47*(4), 411–426.

Good, B. J., & DelVecchio-Good, M. J. (2008). *Indonesia Sakit*: Indonesian Disorders and the Subjective Experience and Interpretive Politics of Contemporary Indonesian Artists. In M.-J. DelVecchio Good, S. Hyde, S. Pinto, & B. J. Good (Eds.), *Postcolonial Disorders* (pp. 62–108). University of California Press.

Ihde, D. (1995). *Postphenomenology: Essays in the Postmodern Context.* Northwestern University Press.

Ihde, D. (2002). *Bodies in Technology* (Vol. 5). University of Minnesota Press.

Jakobson, R. (1956). Two Aspects of Language and Two Types of Aphasic Disturbances. In R. Jakobson (Ed.), *Selected Writings* (Vol. 2, pp. 239–259). Mouton.

Jones, E. (1948). The Theory of Symbolism. In E. Jones (Ed.), *Papers on Pycho-Analysis* (5th ed.). Baillière, Tindall, and Cox.

Klein, M. (1939). The Importance of Symbol-Formation in the Development of the Ego. *International Journal of Psycho-Analysis, 11*, 24–39.

Klein, M. (1952). *Developments in Psycho-Analysis.* Ed. J. Riviere. Hogarth Press.

Klein, M. (1975). *The Psycho-Analysis of Children.* Hogarth.

Kojève, A. (1969). *Introduction to the Reading of Hegel: Lectures on the Phenomenology of Spirit.* Cornell University Press.

Kristeva, J. (1989). *Black Sun: Depression and Melancholia.* Columbia University Press.

Lacan, J. (1953/1996). The Function and Field of Speech and Language in Psychoanalysis. In J. Lacan (Ed.), *Ecrits: The First Complete Edition in English* (pp. 197–268). Trans. B. Fink, H. Fink, and R. Grigg. W. W. Norton & Company.

Lacan, J. (1957/1996). The Instance of the Letter, or Reason since Freud. In J. Lacan (Ed.), *Ecrits: The First Complete Edition in English* (pp. 412–441). Trans. B. Fink, H. Fink, and R. Grigg. W. W. Norton & Company.

Lacan, J. (1981a). *The Seminar of Jacques Lacan: Book XI, the Four Fundamental Concepts of Psychoanalysis.* W. W. Norton & Company.

Lacan, J. (1981b). *The Seminar of Jacques Lacan: Book III, the Psychoses.* W. W. Norton & Company.

Lacan, J. (1988). *The Seminar of Jacques Lacan: Book II, the Ego in Freud's Theory and in the Technique of Psychoanalysis.* W. W. Norton & Company.

Lacan, J. (1996). *Ecrits: The First Complete Edition in English.* Trans. B. Fink, H. Fink, and R. Grigg. W. W. Norton & Company.

Owens, C. (1980). The Allegorical Impulse: Toward a Theory of Postmodernism. *October, 12*, 67–86.

Protevi, J. (2009). *Political Affect: Connecting the Social and the Somatic.* University of Minnesota Press.

Rahimi, S. (2013). The Ego, the Ocular, and the Uncanny: Why Are Metaphors of Vision Central in Accounts of the Uncanny? *The International Journal of Psychoanalysis, 94*(3), 453–476.

Rahimi, S. (2015a). *Meaning, Madness and Political Subjectivity: A Study of Schizophrenia and Culture in Turkey.* Routledge.

Rahimi, S. (2015b). Ghosts, Haunting, and Intergenerational Transmission of Affect: From Cryptonymy to Hauntology. *Psychoanalytic Discourse, 1*(1), 39–45.

Rahimi, S. (2016). Haunted Metaphor, Transmitted Affect: The Pantemporality of Subjective Experience. *Subjectivity, 9*(1), 83–105.

Ricoeur, P. (1975). *The Rule of Metaphor.* Routledge.

Ricoeur, P. (1978). The Metaphorical Process as Cognition, Imagination, and Feeling. *Critical Inquiry* Special Issue on Metaphor, *5*(1), 143–159.

Saussure, F. D. (1959). *Course in General Linguistics.* Trans. W. Baskin. Philosophical Library.

Turner, V. (1982). Images of Anti-Temporality: An Essay in the Anthropology of Experience. *The Harvard Theological Review, 75*(2), 243–265.

Walkerdine, V. (2015). Transmitting Class across Generations. *Theory & Psychology, 25*(2), 167–183.

Walkerdine, V., Olsvold, A., & Rudberg, M. (2013). Researching Embodiment and Intergenerational Trauma Using the Work of Davoine and Gaudilliere: History Walked in the Door. *Subjectivity, 6*(3), 272–297.

Williams, R. (1977). *Marxism and Literature.* Oxford University Press.

Wolfreys, J. (2002). *Victorian Hauntings: Spectrality, Gothic, the Uncanny and Literature.* Palgrave Macmillan.

Woolf, V. (2005). *Selected Works of Virginia Woolf.* Wordsworth Editions.

CHAPTER 4

The Haunted Objects of Desire

Abstract This chapter continues the examination of haunting as a foundational element of the emerging subjective experience, specifically desire and political subjectivity. The discussion here builds on and extends the earlier chapters: Chap. 2 highlighted the ghostly traces left by concrete substance and internal physical experience as they are rendered meaningful through the semiotic transformation of "things" to signifiers; Chap. 3 investigated the role played by high-level linguistic processes of metaphoricity and metonymy in ego formation with specific reference to the notion of death drive; and this chapter examines higher-level psychological processes whereby semiotic and linguistic underpinnings make possible the emergence of desire, which serves in turn as an anchoring point of intentionality and social engagement for the edifice of subjectivity. I use here a clinical example drawn from a psychotic patient's case study to discuss the psychoanalytic notion of objet a, aka the object cause of desire, and its relevance to hauntology by conceptualizing the ghost as a decoupled objet a (of an individual or a group of people, an entire era, or even a historical past as such) which "floats" in the symbolic space because of a culturally unsanctioned termination of the original subject. The orphaned objet a

An earlier version of this chapter has been published in the journal *Ethos* (see Rahimi, 2019).

S. Rahimi, *The Hauntology of Everyday Life*,
https://doi.org/10.1007/978-3-030-78992-3_4

lingers in the shared symbolic space seeking heed from the living—be it in the form of personal haunting or messianic or utopian ideological desire.

Keywords Desire • *Objet petit a* • Subjectivity • Emanet • Lost Object • Object Cause of Desire • Cultural transmission

> *Ghosts come into and pass out of being whether or not man knows of their being, whether he gives much or little thought to them. Because of man, ghosts exist. While man continues as a thinking being and has desires, ghosts will continue to exist.*
> —H. W. Percival

British psychoanalyst Donald Winnicott famously wrote, "should an adult make claims on us for our acceptance of the objectivity of his subjective phenomena, we discern or diagnose madness."[1] As truistic as Winnicott's statement may sound, however, it does not appear to hold in the case of ghostly experiences. Even in our post-industrial societies, we do not rush to diagnose psychosis when an adult claims to have seen or felt the presence of a ghost. There is perhaps something significant about our collective permissiveness when it comes to ghosts and haunting. The majority of us no longer call people who claim speaking to or receiving orders from God prophets and treat them with reverence; we are more likely to suspect psychotic illness, and to convince or force them to undergo medical treatment. But people who claim speaking or receiving messages from ghosts of dead people continue to enjoy popular million-dollar businesses, and TVs and internet sites are littered with highly popular fiction and reality shows built on precisely that claim. It is perhaps also related to this same fact that cultural and even psychological anthropologists pay generally little attention to this real and significant phenomenon. But while in the first casual glance ghosts may appear as insignificant oddities on the peripheries of our anthropological and psychological radars, a second look would swiftly recognize them as much more significant and pervasive, as soon as we realize the ways in which both the phenomenon and the conceptual method we term "hauntology" connect to the most foundational processes in human subjectivity and the psychic apparatus, as we saw in the last chapter. Ghosts and hauntings have the extraordinary capacity of opening on us a window straight to the core of deeply encoded messages that have silently driven our social and political processes throughout history. And hauntology, as an analytic language and as a methodological approach, holds the promise of enabling us to decode the assemblage of our symbolic order in ways that has not been available to us thus far. In this chapter I will address another instance of the ways in which developing a closer understanding and a more cohesive theory of ghosts and haunting would immediately serve the objective of gaining a more robust theory of subjectivity, and a better appreciation of the hauntological nature of subjective experience as such.

OBJET A, THE OBJECT CAUSE OF DESIRE

I will use as my point of entry a story that showcases one of the foundational concepts in hauntology, that is, the semiotic object cause of desire, which, as mentioned earlier, Jacques Lacan has termed *objet a*.[2] The story belongs to Ahmet, whom I met in Turkey many years back during fieldwork on schizophrenia and political subjectivity. Ahmet is a young Turk of Kurdish descent who migrated with his family to Switzerland. He is brought back to Istanbul by his family to be cured from a severe case of *junoon* that the doctors in Europe have not been able to deal with. He is hospitalized in a private psychiatric hospital in Istanbul, diagnosed with Schizophrenia. Ahmet, however, considers himself *majnoon (mecnun*, in Turkish*)*, as do his parents. The word *majnoon* has three simultaneous senses: being afflicted with *junoon* or madness; being struck by the invisible creatures called the *jinn*; and falling madly in love like Majnoon, which is the epithet of the legendary character Qais, who lost his sanity when he was cruelly denied access to his beloved, Layla. Becoming *majnoon* is a common form of madness across the Muslim world. The *jinn* are ghostly creatures living side by side of the human race on earth. They do not usually meddle with our lives and prefer to remain invisible to human eyes, but they are real, as real as you and me, as explicitly stated in the Quran and the Hadith,[3] and confirmed by both Sunni and Shia *ulama*.[4] Once in a while the *jinn* do meddle with humans, with typically severe consequences for humans, specifically insanity or *junoon*. The state of being *majnoon* therefore indicates a juxtaposition of being struck by the *jinn* and being traumatized by the (unfair) loss of a passionately desired love object, a situation of love possession, if you like. I have unpacked the story of Ahmet's love possession elsewhere,[5] and I will not recap that here, but I would like to use his story to address an important feature common to his and many similar cases. That feature is the central role of desire in the most basic patterns of haunting and possession, or to be more precise, the role of *objet a*, formulated as "the object cause of desire,"[6] in the formation of these experiences.

Ahmet, a 27-year-old man, was only 2 years old when his father left the family to work in Switzerland. Two decades later he finally reunited with his father in Switzerland, where before long he fell madly in love with "the Swiss woman." Things did not go too well with the Swiss woman, however, and by the end she did not seem to be as interested in Ahmet as he was in her. She left him, and he spiraled into a psychotic nightmare replete with Islamic characters and symbols, where God and Satan (and their respective underlings, the angels and the *jinn*) collude in an ambiguous dance, conspiring to ruin him in an uncanny space of horror where "nothing is moving in the direction it is supposed to."[7]

Ahmet's story is a strong instance of the deeply intertwined and intricate roles played by national and international politics, religion, and culture in shaping an individual's personality makeup, their inherited patterns of social and political affect, and indeed the psychological workings all the way into their psychotic experiences. Ahmet's and his family's narrative and experience of what has gone wrong in his life are generally formulated on a culturally available semiotic grid, but, more specifically relevant to the present discussion, they are built around the local idiom of love madness, according to which Ahmet is now a *majnoon*, a narrative which is in turn built around the notion of *emanet*, as I will explain below.

Ahmet's story of his affliction begins in a time when "everything was going well," as he repeatedly emphasizes. But that was only "until I met the Swiss woman."

A: [...] then I met a lady, a Swiss lady...We talked, we were nice to each other, chatted ... now in the restaurant, over there, there was one other person. He was Satan [*Şeytan*]...Roki.
S: What was that?
A: Roki. He himself was Satan I mean. I mean a nation worshiping Satan I mean. I mean the Christian world.

The plot is not too thick: Ahmet desires the Swiss woman and he is about to have her, but Satan, represented by a man called Roki who also represents the Christian world, steps between Ahmet and the object of his desire, interrupts his love affair and blocks his attempt at reaching the beloved. "From there on," he says, "unhappiness fell between us." From this point on is also where his storyline becomes more intriguing as things take a mysterious turn that leads eventually to disarray in the very order of the universe.

A: The lady was no good for me. She constantly caused pain, pain after pain; she made me run after her. Since then I've been after the thing I left with her as emanet. If I can get it back from her, then maybe... What I'm trying to say is that maybe millions of people know this, but of course mankind cannot understand it. But when I get it back, then everything will be normal again. It seems that way to me. The world will then return to its normal standard state. Because, as long as I don't have it back I can never find peace. Also, the people around me are also becoming restless and confused. The people that I know and strangers, they are all mixed. I can't see or find the thing that I left with her. That is the reason why I am with the doctors, that I am unwell.

At the center of this turn is a fascinating trope: the lost "thing," the *emanet*, which is what he now seeks in place of the Swiss woman, plays the role of the object cause of desire—*objet a*. In Ahmet's opinion, this lost object is the cause of his madness and so long as the Swiss woman does not return it to him, he will continue to be haunted by her memories and his mind will remain possessed. It is easy and tempting to dismiss Ahmet's formulation of the cause of his love possession as psychotic talk—and his own doctors both in Europe and in Turkey have done exactly that, after all. But what renders his exaltation of the missing object quite difficult to dismiss from such vantage points as cultural psychiatry or psychological anthropology is the clear way in which this formulation recreates powerful local cultural models including both the story of Majnoon and the notion of *junoon*, as well as the prominent Islamic concept of *emanet*. Before I address the notion of *emanet* in more detail, consider the following excerpt where I try to gain a more concrete understanding of what he means by "*emanet*":

S   There is one thing that I can't quite understand and I want to ask you. You said if you get your *emanet* back, then everything will be straightened out.
A   Yes everything will be straightened out.
S   How will everything be straightened out?

A   It all becomes normal then. In my view everything will become normal. But as long as she has not given it back, nothing will come to its
normal state.

S   Yes, so for example what will become normal?

A   Life, life will become normal

S   For instance?

A   For example life, people always do things together, they talk, work,
struggle together. There are factories, I go back to my own work, I
work in the factory, I do this, I do that. Then it's normal. But when
the emanet isn't there, my environment, the surrounding that I face,
is not right, it breaks down. When I say breaks down, my environment gets disordered, and the nation breaks, no one remains peaceful. No, there is nothing, none. All sorrow, depression, pain. It all
piles up on top of each other. But once I get my emanet back, I will
gladly love again, from the depth of my soul. We'll say thanks to
Allah we are saved, we are freed from this emanet thing. After that
everything will be fine, I mean good, I mean really normal...I will
find myself another woman. Understand?

S   Understand.

A   [...] I said, I said I left emanet with you this pack of cigarettes and 10
francs, here, take this and get lost, I don't love you anymore. *Ich liebe
dich nicht*. I don't love you. I'm sorry, I have friends and family, leave
me free from shame and humiliation, and I will be thankful [...] But
that *emanet*, give that to me, that is something very valuable, I mean
it constantly distresses me.

S   Why is it so valuable?

A   When I say valuable [*değerli*], it's because I left it as an *emanet* with
her. I said, one of these days I will be in a hospital, either a hospital
or a prison, I will escape the factory. That was on my mind. Then
from there I ran off to Satan. He took the things I left...

You might be surprised—unless you are a psychoanalyst, perhaps—to
learn that, when at some point Ahmet's family managed to convince the
so-called Swiss woman (who was understandably quite frightened by this
point) to actually come visit Ahmet and give his "*emanet*" back to him,
Ahmet refused to meet with her and said he no longer wanted or needed
his *emanet* back. Of course he then picked up the *emanet* discourse once
again, as soon as the literal possibility of acquiring the "actual" object [a
half pack of cigarettes and a coin of ten Swiss francs] no longer existed.

"They assure themselves," wrote Kristeva in an insightful discussion of the lost objet and its melancholic seekers, "of an inaccessible...ascendancy over the archaic object that thus remains, for themselves and for all others, an enigma and a secret."[8]

What Ahmet is seeking can in fact be understood in both Western psychoanalytic and Eastern philosophical terms, with comparable results. In both traditions the human's capacity of being human, specifically insofar as it is a meaning-making social subject whose sense of self and self-consciousness ultimately depends on the ability to function in a realm of shared symbolic abstractions, depends on "losing" something, the discomforting experience of which loss then becomes the wellspring of motivation: motivation to love, motivation to think, motivation to project ideas (meaning, peace, power—homes, destinations, utopias) onto the future and move forward after that projection. This is what I addressed in some detail in the last chapter. It is in fact this fundamental, existential necessity of the lost object that drives Ahmet to disallow the return of the actual pack of cigarettes and 10 francs—the *emanet* needs to remain lost. Ahmet's problem is not that the emanet continues to remain lost, but that the Swiss woman has refused to accept it for what it means, or even acknowledge its existence, and in doing so, she has effectively subverted the reality and the order of his world, or more importantly, she has foreclosed the possibility of his desire.

I will try to flesh out this confounding idea shortly, but let me connect this account to the question of ghosts and hauntology before doing so. What is haunting Ahmet is not simply that his love is unrequited, but that his object cause of desire is lost in a realm of uncertainty, thus foreclosing the possibility of his world to find its structural equipoise. To make better sense of this we may need to bring back the Islamic notion of *emanet*. The term *emanet* is used frequently in the Quran and holds a special place in Sufi philosophy. Of specific interest to Sufis is the following passage of the Quran, where God describes how and why he ended up leaving the *emanet* with humans:

> Verily We offered the emanet to the heavens and the earth and the mountains, but they refused to bear its load and were frightened by it. Man accepted [to shoulder] the burden. Surely he [Man] is unaware and ignorant![9]

Intriguingly, what exactly this emanet is remains completely obscure and unspoken in the Quran. Humans alone of all of God's creations, according to the Sufi reading of the verse, were "crazy" enough to choose the impossible task of carrying the emanet,[10] because humankind alone is self-conscious and exists on the eternal line of struggle between desire and inhibition. *Emanet* is a part of God, which is left with humans and which commits mankind to an eternal experience of loss which ceaselessly generates a burning desire to reunite with its origin—all earthly love and desire is a manifestation of this desire, and all sorrow and longing is a manifestation of this separation (and hence valuable). Mankind in this account will never arrive at peace until the emanet is returned to its origin, to God, which is possible only in death, or in any case in annihilation of the ego. Now, it is intriguing to note how this account ties almost seamlessly with the Lacanian formulation of desire, and, as we discussed in the last chapter, with the primacy of lack as a prerequisite to the establishment of both meaning and desire, and hence the symbolic order as such. And let's not forget, there can be no means for the subject to distinguish reality from the imaginary before a symbolic order is established and internalized. Or as André Green put it, "it is only in the field of the symbolic that the third term, which is indispensable for the structuring of the psychic process, appears."[11] *Emanet* in this sense can be identified as the source which enables the function of *objet a*. *Objet a*, Lacan insists, should not be mistaken for the desired object, in fact it is not an object: it is the psychic/ semiotic *object cause of desire*, which is injected into (or projected onto, if you prefer) external objects (including signs and other subjects) by the subject, thus turning those into desired objects. "Included in *objet a* is *agalma*, the inestimable treasure that Alcibiades declares is contained in the rustic box the figure of Socrates is to him. But let us note that a minus sign (-) is attributed to it."[12] Think of the minus sign as the fact that, just like *emanet*, this is a special type of object that in fact signifies not a presence but an absence, not a positivity, but a negativity. Just as emanet indicates the absence from God and a separation from the original union (a literal, physical separation, and an "emptiness" that inorganic objects, mountains, rocks and stars do not carry, it is the side effect, if you like, of the capacity to abstract and to symbolize), *objet a* is "the negative of the body."[13] And like *objet a*, *emanet* is located somewhere between reality and fantasy, between symbolic and real, between self and other (keep in mind also earlier discussions on the functions of phoneme and metaphor). It is a part of the real that gets carried by the imaginary, and haunts the symbolic. Or, if you prefer, it is a part of God that humans carry within them. In part for that reason it is that the function of *objet a* can persist, with or without the subject or its desired object. *Objet a* is at once "absolute and inapprehensible, an element necessarily lacking, unsatisfied, impossible, and misconstrued."[14] Because it does not refer to any actual object yet it assumes the semiotic guise of a "thing," it cannot be grasped and described, and for the same reason, it cannot be erased and forgotten either. Ahmet laments repeatedly, "if I could forget that emanet, it would be so nice! If I forget, it will be good for me, but I can't even forget that," or alternatively, "once I get my emanet back… we'll say thanks to Allah we are saved, we are freed from this emanet thing."

A striking feature of Ahmet's story is the clarity with which the entire narrative of his possession is constructed around the function of *emanet/objet a*. Ahmet's object cause of desire has somehow remained "stuck" in limbo, apparently still in the possession of the originally designated object of desire, the Swiss woman. Given the vital role of *objet a* in holding together the fabric of our symbolic system,[15] so long as it is not released to him, the world will be out of order, and he unable to love again:

> when the *emanet* isn't there, my environment, the surrounding that I face, is not right, it breaks down. When I say breaks down, my environment gets disordered, and the nation breaks, no one remains peaceful. No, there is nothing, none. All sorrow, depression, pain. It all piles up on top of each other. But once I get my *emanet* back, I will gladly love again, from the depth of my soul.

Of special interest to me in the account of Ahmet's love possession (*junun*) is the motility of *objet a*. At the base of the idea that Ahmet's *emanet*, a half-empty pack of cigarettes and a 10-franc coin, would exert such extraordinary power over not only his health and well-being but also the order of his universe, lies the implicit assumption that *objet a* is distinct and can in fact be separated not just from the designated object of desire, but also from the desiring subject—albeit at the high cost of the subject's structural disintegration, in the latter case. But how can we actually make sense of such an unusual idea?

The Floating *Objet a*

"As Hegel would have put it," writes Slavoj Zizek, "the excess of the beloved, what, in the beloved, eludes my grasp, is the very place of the inscription of my own desire into the beloved object."[16] This idea speaks to the relation of *objet a* with the object lost to death. Or, to take this back to Lacan, "the work of mourning," he says:

> appears, in a clarification at the same time identical and contrary, as a work that is done to maintain and sustain all these links in detail, in effect, toward the end of restoring the link with the veritable object of the relation, the masked object, the *objet a*.[17]

The subject's main objective in the work of mourning, in other words, is to reconstitute the link with the now-orphaned *objet a*, which it had vested in the now-lost object of desire. Notice again that, as in Ahmet's *emanet*, here too we are speaking of an *objet a* that can survive the death of the object of desire, and needs to be recollected and "brought in," or as Lacan puts it, linked back with. What we are receiving from Lacan is in effect a new reading of mourning and melancholia, which distinguishes between melancholia and successful mourning in terms of the subject's success in retrieving its *objet a*. Ahmet's relentless emphasis on his madness and the fate of his pack of cigarettes and the 10-franc coin finds new justification in this formulation of mourning, given the significant role of *objet a* in holding together the metonymic successions of the symbolic order.

Furthermore, and more directly relevant to the discussion of ghosts and hauntology, the notion of an orphaned or floating *objet a* offers a powerful path forward in a hauntological formulation of ghosts and the experience of haunting. In their discussions of the loss of the object of desire and the ensuing process, both Freud and Lacan have concentrated exclusively on the living person's work of mourning. The conceptualization of *objet a* as a special class of psychosemiotic objects that can persist suspended in the collective space of shared meaning (call it the symbolic space, and think of language or culture), independent of both the desired object and the desiring subject,[18] opens important options in thinking about the nature of ghosts and haunting. It gives us the option, for instance, of thinking of a ghost as the phenomenological manifestation of an orphaned *objet a*—the object cause of desire of a dead subject which persists beyond the subject's demise, encrypted in cultural, linguistic, and semiotic codes and "floating" in the virtual space of collective meanings,

waiting for the right subject to "link" it back to the register of lived experience. Think of Abraham and Torok's notion of the "crypt,"[19] and the
intergenerational transmission of the phantom which is captured in that
crypt and is "transmitted" via the collective space of the symbolic order,
specifically language, from one generation to the next. Little effort is
required to conceptualize the psychosemiotic process whereby an *objet a,*
orphaned due to the (typically abrupt and/or culturally un-processable,
unjustifiable) destruction of its original subject, would remain unprocessed and unfinished, floating in the "limbo" of collectively shared symbolic space until the "right" subject shows up to experience or even own
it (be haunted by it), decode its semiotic content into subjective experience, and possibly even process and resolve it and thus liberate the "ghost"
to move on to the realm of the dead. Keep in mind that, as André Green
emphatically put it, "*objet petit a* is strictly not specularizable," and that,
going back to Lacan's somewhat cryptic words in his seminar on
Identification, the "image" that results from such specularization[20] "is neither the image of the [desired] object nor a representation [of *objet a*], it
is another object which is not the same."[21] The point to take away here is
the clarification that *objet a* is an "object" that exists outside the subject's
"head," yet has no essential ties to any external objects, nor even a specific
image—it can lend itself to various objects, and various acts of
specularization.

In her work on mourning and melancholia, Kristeva too arrives at the
account of ghosts that haunt the living subject through a language that is
dead to them. In her jargon, *objet a* or *emanet* become *La Chose,* the
French version of the Thing, *das Ding.* The melancholic subject, the subject for whom the process of mourning of the loss of the object of desire
has not happened properly, she says,

> experiences difficulty integrating the universal signifying sequence ... the
> dead language they speak ... conceals a Thing buried alive. The latter, how-
> ever, will not be translated in order that it not be betrayed; it shall remain
> walled up within the crypt of the inexpressible affect.[22]

The *emanet* too is an imageless object of a spectral nature in many
senses of the word. It is located somewhere between reality and fantasy,
between symbolic and real, between self and other, and as we saw in the
case of Ahmet, as a non-existent object that needs to be linked-to for symbolic order to be restored. Here again one arrives at the fact that ghosts
and hauntings take place precisely at the interface of the individual and the

collective—and nowhere else: if the experience is exclusively internal and private, it will be psychotic, and if it is exclusively external and collective, it will be metaphoric. It is also thanks to this feature that the *emanet* persists beyond temporality. Because it does not refer to any specific object yet it assumes the semiotic guise of a "thing," it cannot be grasped and described, and for the same reason, it cannot be erased and forgotten either. It functions like a ghost, in other words. And at the core of what I aim to drive home here is that this similarity is neither superficial nor coincidental. They are similar because they are the phenomenological and psychological outcomes of the same set of processes—and what's more, a set of processes that are foundational to the very sense of existence and selfhood and the everyday experience of the social subject.

THE STONE TAPE

In the Christmas of 1972, the British Broadcasting Company aired as its Christmas ghost story a teleplay called *The Stone Tape*,[23] which was destined to become a classic cross-genre cult film—wedding science fiction and ghost lore. *The Stone Tape* captures the story of a team of scientists working on developing new recording technology who, thanks to their wealthy lead scientist, get to move their lab into a renovated Victorian mansion. They soon learn, however, that the mansion has a reputation for being haunted—specifically a large room at the center of the mansion, with stone walls that are remnants of the original building and foundations that date back to the Saxon era. Before long team members experience sounds and visions that confirm the building's reputation. With their scientific expertise, however, they are able to crack the secret of the building's ghosts in a way that locals have not: they discover that the sounds and visions are in fact replays or "projections" of "excessively strong emotions" that have been "encoded" into objects—specifically the ancient stone walls of the haunted room—and hence the film's title. "It's the room! Just the room, itself, nothing else!" insists Peter, the lead scientist:

> There's no ghost [everybody objects]. OK, try this for science: the room holds an image, and when people go in they pick it up. What you hear, or what you see, is inside your own brain. That'd be why the sounds don't echo and why we can't locate them. That'll be why they don't record on our machines... Don't you get it yet? It must act like a recording. Fixed in the floor and the walls. Right in the substance of them a trace of what happened there. And we pick it up. We act as detectors, recorders, amplifiers.

Even though the desires and emotions of the dead are encrypted into the environment, people who step into the room do not "sense" the recordings to the same degree. While Jill (who is a medium outside of her day job as a scientist) and one other team member both hear and see the screaming ghost, Peter and some others can only hear the screams, and still others do not see or hear anything. Peter says of one man who cannot hear or see the screaming ghost: "He's ghost proof. Like color blind!"

Interestingly, *The Stone Tapes* was inspired by the writings of T.C. Lethbridge, a British anthropologist-turned-parapsychologist. Drawing analogy from his contemporary TV broadcasting technology, Lethbridge had theorized ghosts sighted by living individuals as "pictures projected by somebody else," through a process in which the viewer is "nothing more than the receiving set."[24] The ghost, in this way, can be understood as a message inscribed in an invisible signal originating from a dying person and suspended in air or some as-yet-unknown medium, which is then reproduced as spectral visions or even somatic experiences by "the sensitive's mind."[25] Ghosts, he wrote, can be given "some rudimentary existence," or "some kind of substance," which, he was quick to qualify, "is created by thought."[26] Admittedly, the idea of some rudimentary existence or some kind of substance created by thought comes as close as any definition that I know to the idea of "spectrality."

In a basic sense, when I say I am haunted by another subject's ghost, unless I am speaking metaphorically, I am saying my subjectivity is frequented by an other's subjectivity. I am, in other words, conveying a process in which the other's *objet a* has substituted mine or is incorporated into mine in a discernible way, in effect imprinting the dead person's desire upon my own. Insofar as "subjectivity" can be understood as an apparatus the function of which is seeking to attain the "lost" object of desire, when I am haunted, I am taken over (possessed) by the subjectivity that was an other's. In Abraham and Torok's words, "the phantom's periodic and compulsive return lies beyond the scope of symptom formation in the sense of a return of the repressed; it works like a ventriloquist, like a stranger within the subject's own mental topography."[27]

It is no coincidence that the single most common theme in our lore and our associations to haunting is that of the spectral remainder of a dead person that has stayed back to haunt, in a quest to have an unfulfilled desire of the dead subject fulfilled through the living. Ghosts, says Dr. James Harvey, the "ghost psychiatrist" in the 1995 popular movie *Casper*, "are known for haunting us. My question is, what is haunting them? It's a lack of resolution! Ghosts are simply spirits without resolution, with unfinished business. And it's my job to find out what that is." The highly successful American TV series *Ghost Whisperer*, which ran on the CBS channel for over five years,[28] was constructed entirely around the basic theme of wandering ghosts of dead subjects in need of a surrogate subject to manage their unfinished desires. Melinda Gordon, the main character (acted by Jennifer Love Hewitt), is "cursed" by her sensitivity to picking up ghosts' presence where others are just too thick or insensitive ("ghost proof," as *The Stone Tape*'s Peter would put it) to perceive them. She tries in each episode to help another ghost get his or her dead subject's unfulfilled desires processed so that they can move on to their next natural order of existence as dead subjects. Once there is no longer a desire in need of fulfillment, the wandering *objet a* automatically dissolves and disappears, it "goes away."

As I have pointed out earlier, one important aspect of theorizing ghosts and haunting from a hauntological point of view, that is, in terms of *objet a*, is that in this way haunting is formulated as a phenomenon bound to collective processes, specifically through the symbolic systems of meaning. Remember Ahmet's lament in describing what has been affected by the loss of his emanet:

A   For example life, people always do things together, they talk, work, struggle together. There are factories, I go back to my own work, I work in the factory, I do this, I do that. Then it's normal. But when the emanet isn't there, my environment, the surrounding that I face, is not right, it breaks down. When I say breaks down, my environment gets disordered, and the nation breaks, no one remains peaceful.

This is why ghosts act or speak in terms of a local cultural logic which may not be easily decoded cross-culturally. When an individual life is terminated, it is the local cultural logic that determines whether that subjectivity has been extinguished appropriately and whether the lost subjects' *objet a* shall be reintegrated back within the collective space, or if that termination has been unjust, untimely or otherwise inappropriate, in which case an *objet a* may be incapable of reabsorption into the collective space, and may remain as a dis-embodied object cause of desire which will stay dormant (or encrypted, to use Abraham and Torok's terminology) in the collective space of language and cultural memory. Think of the floating bits of genetic code we call viruses, and the way they can remain dormant for long periods of time until they encounter and "possess" the living body of a suitable host, which will then serve as a vehicle through which the virus manages to express and complete its genetic desire. "Language itself becomes haunted," writes Gabriele Schwab, who then lists a range of semiotic tropes that can contain the lost signification, including metaphors, metonymies, homophonies, homonymies, puns, semantic ambiguities, malapropisms, anagrams, rebuses and other such tropes that "combine concealment and revelation."[29] The dormant object cause of desire can then turn into a "ghost" if and when a correctly positioned subject reacts to it, adopts it, and brings back to the social arena the orphaned *objet a*. Like geological "hotspots" in the arena of continental drift, "the sensitives" are first to react to the forces repressed by conflicting tectonic encounters, and they become volcanic vents for the pressure of the orphaned *objet a*. To make things yet more interesting, consider also that an orphaned *objet a* does not need to be literally born of an individual death: it can be created in the process of mass destruction born out of large-scale atrocities committed in political turmoil, genocides, or even natural disasters such as massive earthquakes or tsunamis as many report from around the world. We may have lacked a good theoretical framework to explain how or why, but we have nonetheless noticed that throughout history waves of ghost sightings and hauntings have often followed such unexpected and unaccepted mass atrocities and mass destructions.[30]

The "wrongful death" in these situations may or may not be traceable back to specific individuals, and the ghosts that haunt the survivors may or may not appear known or familiar to them.[31] That the ghosts emerging out of collective atrocities and grief are no longer easily tied to individual desires points the way back to the sociopolitical relevance of haunting and the significance of theorizing ghosts from a hauntological point of view. "Being with" specters, says Derrida, calls on "a politics of memory, of inheritance, and of generations"[32] which stretches well beyond the simple algorithms of psychological genealogy. Like ghost encounters and individual hauntings, the resurfacing of historical ghosts and the haunting of living societies by otherwise forgotten (read repressed, if you prefer) discourses and affective patterns of past generations are simultaneously individual psychological phenomena insofar as the effect can be identified at the individual affective level, and sociopolitical processes with broad collective impact and manifestations. It is most certainly not a "random" effect that certain groups of individuals, certain cultural environments or certain historical periods are more prone to "picking up" and even enacting a specific dormant often obscured set of desires of the presumed-dead pasts of their history. And it is perhaps time for our social and human sciences to take note of this problem and realize the need for understanding it. And it is also time for us to take note of the uniquely "hauntological" logic that underlies the vast range of phenomena from broad sociopolitical movements and events to individual everyday affects, perceptions, and decision making.

NOTES

1. Winnicott, 1953, p. 96.
2. The term, often read "*objet petit-a*" literally means "object little-a," with "a" standing for *autre* (other) in French and therefore technically translatable as "object o" or "object little-o." Lacan, however, has famously requested of his readers to avoid translating this term and for it to be used in its original French form, "thus acquiring the status of an algebraic sign" (Lacan, 1977, p. xi). Respecting his advice, I have chosen to present the term as *objet a* throughout this book.
3. Second in significance only to the Quran, the Hadith comprise a body of narratives recounting the words, actions, and habits of prophet Muhammad, his direct heirs, and, for the Shia, 12 of his descendants.
4. Literally "the learned ones," ulama are scholars recognized as main authorities of reference in questions of Islamic tradition, hermeneutics, and jurisprudence.
5. Fragments of Ahmet's story presented here are drawn from my 2015 book, *Meaning, Madness and Political Subjectivity* (see pp. 155–198). To gain a more meaningful appreciation of his intricate story, I strongly recommend reading the full case analysis.
6. See for instance Lacan, 1981, or Žižek, 1992.
7. This and following excerpts are quoted from Rahimi, 2015, pp. 155–198.
8. Kristeva, 1989, p. 64.
9. The Quran, Ch. 33, Verse 72.
10. Divan of Hafez, Ghazal 338: The heavens were too weak to shoulder the load of emanet / So the lot fell upon me, the crazy one (translation mine)
11. Green, 1966, p. 17.
12. Lacan, 1957, p. 699.
13. Dosse, 1997, p. 243.
14. Manon, 2012, p. 40.
15. The anchoring work of *les points de capiton*, according to Lacan, is possible due to the function of *objet a*. "It is the loss of *objet petit a* as an object that provokes desire and as an object of desire per se that both makes the subject speak and is that about which he will speak, while always eluding him" (Dosse, 1997, p. 244).

16. Žižek, 2006, pp. 355–356.
17. Lacan, 2004, p. 387.
18. *"Objet a* is a lost object, an object that the subject separates itself from in order to constitute itself as a desiring subject" (McGowan, 2012, p.6).
19. Abraham and Torok, 1994.
20. In the process of infant's identification with the image in mirror, for instance.
21. Green, 1966, p. 28.
22. Kristeva, 1989, p. 53.
23. British Broadcasting Corporation, 1972.
24. Lethbridge, 1961, p. 9.
25. Lethbridge, 1961, p. 24.
26. Lethbridge, 1961, p. 46.
27. Abraham and Torok, 1994, p. 173.
28. Dishner and Love Hewitt, 2005–2010.
29. Schwab, 2010, p. 54.
30. See for instance Good, 2015; Good and DelVecchio-Good; 2008; Goulding, 2017; Parry, 2017; Varley et al., 2012.
31. See for instance Leshkowich, 2008.
32. Derrida, 1994, p. xviii.

References

Abraham, N., & Torok, M. (1994). *The Shell and the Kernel: Renewals of Psychoanalysis* (Vol. 1). Trans. N. T. Rand. University of Chicago Press.

British Broadcasting Corporation. (1972). *The Stone Tape.* BBC2 Studio.

Derrida, J. (1994). *Specters of Marx: The State of the Debt, the Work of Mourning, and the New International.* Trans. P. Kamuf. Routledge.

Dishner, J., & Love Hewitt, J. (Producers) (2005–2010). *Ghost Whisperer.* CBS Paramount Network Television.

Dosse, F. (1997). *History of Structuralism: The Rising Sign, 1945–1966* (Vol. 1). University of Minnesota Press.

Good, B. J. (2015). Haunted by Aceh: Specters of Violence in Post-Suharto Indonesia. In D. E. Hinton & A. L. Hinton (Eds.), *Genocide and Mass Violence: Memory, Symptom, and Recovery* (pp. 58–82). Cambridge University Press.

Good, B. J., & DelVecchio-Good, M. J. (2008). *Indonesia Sakit:* Indonesian Disorders and the Subjective Experience and Interpretive Politics of Contemporary Indonesian Artists. In M.-J. DelVecchio Good, S. Hyde, S. Pinto, & B. J. Good (Eds.), *Postcolonial Disorders* (pp. 62–108). University of California Press.

Goulding, C. (2017). Living with Ghosts, Living Otherwise. In *(Re) Constructing Memory: Education, Identity, and Conflict* (pp. 241–268). Sense Publishers.

Green, A. (1966). L'objet (a) de J. Lacan, sa logique et la théorie freudienne. *Cahiers pour l'analyse, 3*, 15–37.

Kristeva, J. (1989). *Black Sun: Depression and Melancholia*. Columbia University Press.

Lacan, J. (1957/1996). The Instance of the Letter, or Reason Since Freud. In J. Lacan (Ed.), *Ecrits: The First Complete Edition in English* (pp. 412–441). W. W. Norton & Company.

Lacan, J. (1977). *Ecrits: A Selection*. Trans. A. Sheridan. Tavistock.

Lacan, J. (1981). *The Seminar of Jacques Lacan: Book XI, the Four Fundamental Concepts of Psychoanalysis*. W. W. Norton & Company.

Lacan, J. (2004). *Le Seminaire de Jacques Lacan, Livre X: L'Angoisse*. Editions de Seuil.

Leshkowich, A. M. (2008). Wandering Ghosts of Late Socialism: Conflict, Metaphor, and Memory in a Southern Vietnamese Marketplace. *The Journal of Asian Studies, 67*(1), 5–41.

Lethbridge, T. C. (1961). *Ghost and Goul*. Routledge and K. Paul.

Manon, H. S. (2012). Partition and Desire in the Films of Joseph H. Lewis. In G. Ryodes (Ed.), *The Films of Joseph H. Lewis* (pp. 38–61). Wayne University Press.

McGowan, T. (2012). *The Real Gaze: Film Theory After Lacan*. SUNY Press.

Parry, R. L. (2017). *Ghosts of the Tsunami: Death and Life in Japan's Disaster Zone*. MCD.

Rahimi, S. (2015). *Meaning, Madness and Political Subjectivity: A Study of Schizophrenia and Culture in Turkey*. Routledge.

Rahimi, S. (2019). Specularizing the Object Cause of Desire of the Dead Other: A Ghost Story. *Ethos, 47*(4), 427–439.

Schwab, G. (2010). *Haunting Legacies: Violent Histories and Transgenerational Trauma*. Columbia University Press.

Varley, E., Isaranuwatchai, W., & Coyte, P. C. (2012). Ocean Waves and Roadside Spirits: Thai Health Service providers' Post-Tsunami Psychosocial Health. *Disasters, 36*(4), 656–675.

Winnicott, D. W. (1953). Transitional Objects and Transitional Phenomena: A Study of the First Not-Me Possession. *International Journal of Psycho-Analysis, 34*, 89–97.

Žižek, S. (1992). *Looking Awry: An Introduction to Jacques Lacan through Popular Culture*. MIT press.

Žižek, S. (2006). *The Parallax View*. MIT Press.

CHAPTER 5

Hauntology sans Exorcism, from Justice to Networked Subjectivities

Abstract In this closing chapter I briefly recap the book's basic formulation of the different layers of abstraction via which original lifeless substance is transformed and transmitted into conscious communication of symbolic representations, highlighting the ubiquity with which the hauntogenic process appears to be at work across diverse developmental paths to human subjectivity. I then indicate two significant implications of hauntological understanding of everyday life: the question of justice, and the future of subjectivity. Given that any dominant discourse and any regime of truth have to establish a systemic repression of other meanings in order to become the dominant discourse or the regime of truth, a hauntological point of view understands justice as an expression of lost voices. A hauntology of everyday life is not meant to exorcise the everyday life or to heal it, nor does it pursue a specific political order or have in mind an attainable and defined formulation of justice. Hauntology upsets the political order and the normative notion of justice as an end attainable through law, and it is through such destabilization, of the law, the language, and the regime of truth as such, that justice emerges as an articulation of lost meanings. The chapter and this book end on a brief discussion of the relevance of hauntological theory to theorizing the emerging forms of subjectivity and subjective experience, specifically the already-in-place networked subjectivity, but also perhaps the capacity to anticipate and theorize the possibility of artificial subjectivity, subjectivity that depends on and is contained within the synthetic networks of artificial agents

© The Author(s), under exclusive license to Springer Nature Switzerland AG 2021
S. Rahimi, *The Hauntology of Everyday Life*,
https://doi.org/10.1007/978-3-030-78992-3_5

of sensing, perceiving, and conceptualizing the physical reality and icating that information via super-compact symbolic forms.

Keywords Justice • Law • Exorcism • Regimes of truth • Networked subjectivity • Artificial subjectivity

> *The more enlightened our houses are, the more their walls ooze ghosts.*
> —Italo Calvino
>
> *I think of ghosts and haunting as just being alert. If you're really alert, then you see the life that exists beyond the life that is on top. It's not spooky necessarily--might be--but it doesn't have to be. It's something I relish rather than run from.*
> —Toni Morrison

In a paper published in the journal *Astronomy and Astrophysics*, an international team of astrophysicists from the Keck Observatory report their intriguing observation that a star named PG 1610+062 has been hurled across the Milky Way galaxy in a slingshot move around the gravitational core of a black hole—an event challenging all of astronomy's familiar ejection mechanisms.[1] I have no intention of committing the common error of a direct comparison across such diverse areas of understanding, but the idea of a black hole and its gravitational force offers a great analogy for the function of the void created through the process of loss frequently addressed in this book, whereby, as Hegel put it, substance becomes subject, and the "pure simple negativity" that is born of that process.[2] Not unlike the black hole around which a star was slingshot, *objet a* serves as "a pivot made of nothing" in the physics of symbolic semiosis. Even though it can best be described as the imaginary location of a lack projected onto an external object, *objet a* is able to produce an immense amount of psychic gravity around which desire can then "sling" and find its way back to the subject, creating the effect of an anchor point within the otherwise unraveling fabric of a system of meanings—what Lacan calls a *point de capiton*. Unlike the Milky Way's black hole story which depicts an uncommon event, however, the slingshotting of desire around a pivot created by *objet a* needs to be understood as a basic and recurrent mechanism that constitutes points of anchorage that hold together the structure of meaning, make possible the outward expression of desire, and beget subjective temporality. Jacques Lacan produced substantive elaborations on the mechanisms involved in the creation and the role of *objet a*, and even though especially toward the end of his life he developed a renewed interest in the dynamics and the implications of *objet a*, it would be safe to say he has left us with only the beginnings of a full account of the generativity of trauma, the apparatus that transforms loss into meaning, and more importantly, the microdynamics of subjective experience or social affect. What I have aimed to highlight here in terms of a hauntology of everyday life is simply the pragmatic everyday relevance of such a theory, and the urgent need for this line of investigation. In the progressive stages of abstraction from pure materiality of lifeless substance to the abstract virtuality of networked subjectivity, with each increment of abstraction required to form a new register of representation comes an inevitable amount of "loss," as something of the original "thing/object" fails to fully translate into the new register. That loss is subsequently incorporated in the new system as spectrality, an absent presence, a negativity. But the absent presence is not inert, it engages the dynamics of representation as a ghost, and it causes substantial effect. And it is not the unfamiliarity, but the ubiquity of this basic process that we need to be astounded by. As Toni Morrison put it, "if you're really alert, then you see the life that exists beyond the life that is on top. It's not spooky necessarily--might be--but it doesn't have to be."[3]

Consider the psychoanalytic object relational model of development, in which each "giving up" of bits and pieces of an original register in order to arrive at the next more distinct and better defined unitary ego leaves a trace in what remains to be a part of the emerging self. This applies to all "lost" objects, be it the physical body of the mother lost gradually through fetal development and finally at birth, or the breast, or the numerous internal experiences later "lost" to symbolization. These various objects gradually become externalized and no longer experienced by the maturing ego as parts of itself, but each and all of them have left traces carved into the complex layers that form the resulting subject. Each object lost/ceded in each stage from the materiality of physical experience to the phenomenality of sensual and affective perception to the virtuality of symbolic and cognitive experience leaves its own respective type of trace on the subject. This is the generativity of trauma. This is a story of loss serving as "work," in the Hegelian sense of *work*: as it destroys something to the infant, it serves to propel the infant toward subjecthood. One could read Hegel's formulation of the role of work in creating the very subjectivity of the subject as if he was writing about the role of ceding in the object relational development of the infant's ego. It is, according to Hegel, in the act of *negating* physical reality (think of negating the original form of a rock to produce a sculpture), that an individual *creates* his or her subjectivity. This is captured perhaps best in Alexander Kojéve's reading of Hegel, who emphasizes, "negating action is not purely destructive, for if action destroys an objective reality...it creates in its place, in and by that very destruction, a subjective reality."[4]

The ubiquity with which the hauntogenic process appears to be at work across diverse developmental paths to human subjectivity is the single most convincing argument for and evidence of the need for a coherent hauntological theory of subjectivity and subjective experience. If this book has been able to drive this single point home, then it has succeeded to do what it was meant to. A hauntology of everyday life is not meant to exorcise the everyday life or to heal it, nor does it pursue a specific political order or have in mind an attainable and defined formulation of justice. As a matter of fact, hauntology upsets the political order and the normative notion of justice as an end attainable through law. Just as the ghost "upsets all calculations, interests, and capital,"[5] hauntology upsets the order of things and subverts the very regime of truth within which justice may have been sought and defined. Hauntology upsets the political order of meaning as it upsets the foundational binaries that underlie what we understand as modern thought. It undermines the epistemological structure on which our knowledge and our order of power are constructed. By driving home the simple fact that any dominant discourse and any regime of truth in order to be a dominant discourse or to become the regime of truth, has to establish a systemic repression of other meanings, hauntology becomes a de facto revolutionary theory. But not a revolution seeking to replace a dominant order with another, it becomes a theory of eternal revolution, if you like, since every meaning, every order, and every representation is haunted by that which it has failed or refused to represent, that which is not meant, that which is not specularized, and which is therefore a potential victim in need of a voice, and a potential contender for a regime of its own. Justice in this sense then belongs to the order of imaginary, justice belongs to the same order of things as did *emanet* and *objet a*. Justice resides outside the law. While the law is constructed and hence deconstructable, justice is not constructed and hence it is not deconstructable. Justice can only be approached, never reached, as a form of liberation of that which has been suppressed and yet has survived the suppression and

Lastly, I would like to end this book by referring back to a brief discussion in Chap. 3 concerning the relevance and implications of hauntology for the emerging modes of experience including the notion of networked subjectivity and even artificial subjectivity. Consider the rapid transition we are currently witnessing, the transition of social and personal interactions from the arena of physical presence to the domain of virtual presence and virtual interactions. Note that this transition exemplifies another "step" in what I had suggested earlier as a series of steps or stages of augmented abstraction—though with different implications, Jean Beaudrillard's layers of simulacra may offer a useful point of orientation here.[16] Not only much of what traditionally took place in the physical space, such as shopping, reading the newspaper, socializing with friends and speaking to strangers has transitioned into cyberspace, but even processes that were already "abstract" such as speech, film, texts and so on, have now acquired further levels of abstraction with new realities, so that textuality has been replaced by hypertextuality, long-lasting TV series have become bingeable, facial gestures and body language have been replaced by emoticons and emojis, and much more. While none of this may sound particularly new or intriguing, I am listing them to call your attention to two points: first, as the basic paradigm and parameters of subjectivity and certainly of social subjectivity have drastically shifted, the obvious question rises as to what the impacts of this new paradigm of subjective experience may be, for the individual and for the society—what mechanisms will drive those, and what dynamics can we expect to emerge? What does/will this mean for the dynamics of desire, structures of feelings, and patterns of affect—subjective features that determine not simply our individual experience, but also our consumption patterns, our political orientations and ideological moorings, not to mention the type of "alternative facts" we end up perceiving the world through. Needless to say, reality is as always ahead of us, as the pressing questions and bewilderment caused by the American social and political mayhem during the last five or six years confirm. Real life has gone well ahead of our theories to show us what it really looks like when a society's dominant regime of truth falls apart and alternative truths come out to openly compete for power, leaving little room for doubt that the epistemologies of old are no longer capable of explaining, much less determining or even containing the "reality" of our age. These are fascinating and powerful events a detailed unpacking of which I have to leave to a future occasion, but I bring this up simply to state that hauntology in fact offers a most powerful tool for engaging these new realities, insofar as it comes prepared for understanding the spectrality of desire, the ex-centricity of the networked subject, and the endless nature of metonymic deferment. And perhaps more importantly, hauntology would aptly start by asking the question of what is lost in the transition of so much of our everyday experience from the physical space to the virtual, and what modalities of desire may that loss give rise to—a question hardly conceivable outside the hauntological formulation of loss and desire, and well positioned to also point the way toward a conceptualization of what a conscious artificial agent may desire.

NOTES

1. Irrgang et al., 2019, see also a brief report on this paper at Keck Observatory's website: https://keckobservatory.org/blackhole-slingshot/
2. Hegel describes "Spirit" (*Geist*) as substance that has become subject, and emphasizes: "as subject, substance is pure simple negativity" (Hegel, 2018, p. 11).
3. Morrison, 2004.
4. Kojève, 1969, p. 4.
5. Derrida, 1994, p. 171.
6. Derrida, 1990, p. 242.
7. Calvino, 1987, p. 19
8. Colin Davis (2013) has written a wonderful examination of this difference which I recommend to anybody interested in the topic. The following discussion includes excerpts from an article of mine published earlier in *Psychoanalytic Discourse* (Rahimi, 2015).
9. Derrida, 1986, p. xix.
10. Abraham and Torok, 1994, p. 159.
11. Derrida, 1994, p. 150.
12. Derrida and Stiegler, 1996, p. 131, quoted in Davis, 2007, p. 75.
13. Rashkin, 1992, p. 12.
14. Davis, 2013, p. 58.
15. Rodriguez, 2001, p. 190.
16. Baudrillard, 1994.

REFERENCES

Abraham, N., & Torok, M. (1994). *The Shell and the Kernel: Renewals of Psychoanalysis* (Vol. 1). Trans. N. T. Rand. Chicago University of Chicago Press.

Baudrillard, J. (1994). *Simulacra and Simulation*. University of Michigan Press.

Calvino, I. (1987). *The Uses of Literature*. Harcourt Brace.

Davis, C. (2007). *Haunted Subjects: Deconstruction, Psychoanalysis and the Return of the Dead*. Palgrave Macmillan.

Davis, C. (2013). *Etats Présent*: Hauntology, Spectres, and Phantoms. In M. del Pilar Blanco & E. Peeren (Eds.), *The Spectralities Reader: Ghosts and Haunting in Contemporary Cultural Theory*. Bloomsbury.

Derrida, J. (1986). *Fors: The Anglish Words of Nicolas Abraham and Maria Torok*. Trans. B. Johnson. Foreword to N. Abraham and M. Torok, *The Wolf Man's Magic Word: A Cryptonymy*. University of Minnesota.

Derrida, J. (1990). Force of Law: The "Mystical Foundation of Authority". *Cardozo Law Review, 11*(5/6), 919–1045.

Derrida, J. (1994). *Specters of Marx: The State of the Debt, the Work of Mourning, and the New International*. Trans. P. Kamuf. Routledge.

Derrida, J., & Stiegler, B. (1996). *Echographies: De la Television*. Galilée / Institut national de l'audiovisuel.

Hegel, G.W.F. (2018). *The Phenomenology of Spirit: Translated with Introduction and Commentary*. Ed./Trans. M. Inwood. Oxford University Press.

Irrgang, A., Geier, S., Heber, U., Kupfer, T., & Fürst, F. (2019). PG 1610+062: A Runaway B Star Challenging Classical Ejection Mechanisms. *Astronomy & Astrophysics, 628*, L5. Online Access: https://www.aanda.org/articles/aa/full_html/2019/08/aa35429-19/aa35429-19.html

Kojève, A. (1969). *Introduction to the Reading of Hegel: Lectures on the Phenomenology of Spirit*. Cornell University Press.

Morrison, T. (2004). *Toni Morrison's 'Good' Ghosts* [Radio Broadcast]. *NPR Morning Edition* Interview Broadcast on September 20, 2004. Audio and Transcript Available Online: https://www.npr.org/transcripts/3912464

Rahimi, S. (2015). Ghosts, Haunting, and Intergenerational Transmission of Affect: From Cryptonymy to Hauntology. *Psychoanalytic Discourse, 1*(1), 39–45.

Rashkin, E. (1992). *Family Secrets and the Psychoanalysis of Narrative*. Princeton University Press.

Rodriguez, S. (2001). Subject. In H. Glowinski, Z. M. Marks, & S. Murphy (Eds.), *A Compendium of Lacanian Terms* (pp. 192–197). Free Association Books.

CHAPTER 6

Epilogue by Michael M.J. Fischer: Hauntology's Genesis, Catacoustics, and Future Shadows

Abstract Hauntology has gone through three major historical formations indexed by dreamwork, electronic music, and algorithmic simulacra. Rahimi introduces the first with: a story of a mentally disturbed man as a kind of *midrash* (often a story mode of biblical or qur'anic interpretation); the second with the analogy of justice as a slingshot around a black hole; and the third with an invocation of emergent cyberworlds and virtual reality as new forms of power relations depending less on information than on data and simulacra. Hauntology itself is the undoing of all ontology, all singularities, all claims to singular origins; of singular sovereignties, of the unified self, and of European philosophy as a restricted language game. Behind every claim of "how things are" lie shadows, ghosts, temporary suppressions of alternatives and contestations in the rich possibilities of life, history, politics, justice, and desire. The first horizon, of psychoanalysis before 1970, is evoked in the rich metaphorical languages drawn from Genesis, the Qur'an, the poetry of Hafiz, and the seventeenth-century Golem at the dawn of the scientific revolution. The horizon of the 1970s is evoked through electronic music and sampling in popular music, playing upon the sonic (blue note) difference between ontology and hauntology. The music scene in England in particular,

Michael M.J. Fischer is Andrew W. Mellon Professor in the Humanities, and Professor of Anthropology and Science and Technology Studies at the Massachusetts Institute of Technology (MIT).

© The Author(s), under exclusive license to Springer Nature Switzerland AG 2021
S. Rahimi, *The Hauntology of Everyday Life*,
https://doi.org/10.1007/978-3-030-78992-3_6

beginning with the Thatcher-Reagan era articulated a sense that the past as cultural resource was nearing exhaustion, that all past senses of the future were being foreclosed, and that the new digital worlds threatened to be subject to neoliberal manipulation as datafication and gamification became tools of replacing the welfare state and social democracy. The emergent third horizon of contemporary cyberworlds is one of contending with "operational images" (legible to machines more than to humans), "modeling," and self-generating digital and biological networks, over which we need to take control choreographically, to produce decolonial pluri-worlds and what Andean nations (among other places) are producing under the banners of, in Quechua, *sumak kawsay* (Spanish, *buen Vivir;* English: good or beautiful life). These are not mere slogans but have brought an indigenous president to power in Bolivia, changed the terms of politics in Peru, and are being struggled over in decentralized health care in Columbia, as well as municipal experiments in Barcelona. All are struggles in process, all are haunted by pasts. These pasts and hauntologies may not operate as they have in the past.

Keywords Hauntology • Memory disorders • Electronic music and sampling • Gamification and datafication • Pluri-culturalism • Social democracy and buen vivir (sumak kawsay) • Hauntogenesis • Golems and artificial intelligence (AI) • Operational images and simulacra • Dreamwork and algorithms

DERRIDA: THE DEPOSIT (*EMANET*) AND THE ALPHABET OF TRUTH (*EMET*), GENESIS OF HAUNTOLOGY

haunting is historical ... but not dated. always more than one.
—Derrida, *Specters of Marx*

In his beautiful midrash, Sadeq Rahimi tells us the story of Ahmet, a young majnoon (a person crazy for an elusive object of desire), who speaks in tongues or through a symbolic order fractured by an imaginary, about which he is both lucid and unaware. He seemingly is unaware that he is recycling a Qur'anic, Sufi, and Jewish set of ideas. He is, we might say, *haunted* by a semiotic discourse. He feels that this discourse expresses his deepest feelings. And although he insists that he needs the packet of cigarettes and ten francs that he left with a Swiss woman, Sadeq Rahimi suggests that we understand this metaphorically and psycho-dynamically as wanting back his deposit (Turkish *emanet,* Persian/Arabic *amanat,*

Hebrew *amanah*). *Emanet,* Rahimi reminds us, appears in the Qur'an, verse 33:72, which Rahimi further unpacks with a verse of the Persian poet Hafez (Ghazal 338) in which only humans are "crazy enough" (*divaneh* or *majnoon,* in love with God enough) to choose the impossible task of carrying the *emanet* which God wishes to deposit with them.

Any reader of the bible (Hebrew, *torah*) will recognize this as a repetition of the story of Moses at Mt. Sinai. Even as a telephone game version (slightly muddled in transmission), nonetheless the story is potent, legible across variants, and psycho-dynamically of value to Ahmet. In the bible, it is the children of Israel who are the only ones God can find to take up his commandments. More importantly, the story is connected with the breaking of the first set of tablets, repeated in Islam through the theological understanding that the Qur'an is but a transcript, an unordered set of revelations, recited first to companions, and only later written down, and ordered by length. The Qur'anic text (however sacred the Arabic is considered) is but a *transcript* in human language of the divine language beyond full human comprehension of the Qur'an in heaven. In both cases, the moral is that humans are in charge of their own interpretive fates. The task is to interpret without letting moral and psychological worlds become untethered and amoral, corrupt, and mere power games. The task is not mere intellectual play (justice in principle) but with social justice in practice.

Sigmund Freud would be tickled. Or rather, Slavoj Zizek, the Lacanian exegete, would be tickled on Freud's behalf. Freud probably would be irritated to be recalled into Jewish traditions he tried to sublimate, but in whose loops of semiotic-desire he, like Ahmet, is always already trapped. Hafiz, as Rahimi hints, elaborates on the diversions in Shiraz's taverns, (wine, entrancements) that metaphorize the dissolution of the big Self: the illusion of a rational Ich (ego), the irrational das Es (id), and the repressive norms of the Über-Ich (super-ego) and freedom from society's repressions.

Ahmet or Ahmad, is a variant of the name Mohammad, and means "the praiseworthy." Mohammad is the "seal" (the last) of the many prophets recognized in Islam, the first of whom was Adam, made from earth and imbued with living breath. He is thus also the seal (certifying stamp) of *haq,* truth. Might *emanet* be also a slippage (of either the Freudian or Lacanian sort), a misprison (à la Harold Bloom) of the Hebrew *emet?* *Emet* means truth or life. The two words are not philologically related, but it is his life, his truth, his deposit, that Ahmet wants back, not its substitutes, its deferrals, its floating placeholders, or its cigarettes and francs.

Emet is what the sixteenth-century Marahal, Rabbi Judah Loew ben Bezalel, of Prague, inscribed on the forehead of the golem to animate it; and then would erase the first letter to de-animate it (*met,* "dead"), either for the sabbath or when it might go out of control. The golem, although the word is used only once in the torah to mean "the unformed," has a long history of extension and contraction. The contemporary variant is what computer scientists call AI (artificial intelligence), with aspirations to download the brain into silicon, create avatars, intelligent robots, smart cities, and informated environments. Indeed Zizek jokes, why not allow computational machines to vote for us, since soon our quantified selves, our preferences (tallied continuously by Amazon), and interests (tallied by Google) will make machines know us better than we can ourselves (and will save needless anxiety, fretting, and depression about who to vote for among unpalatable choices, or what policies to advocate for in increasing double-bind choices of conflicting imperatives). We thus already have multiple ghost selves operating in the machines (networks, servers, data banks) beyond our ken. The Marahal's golem was an iRobot-like servant for the Marahal, a protective fantasy for a Jewish community repeatedly subjected to pogroms, and a cautionary figure regarding man's hubris in trying to compete with God in creation (as one leaves a flaw in a carpet to show this is not one's intent and that perfection is not attained). But, perhaps most interestingly and proleptically, it was created at the beginning of the scientific revolution at the central European (Prague) court of Rudolph II, at the time of Tycho Brahe, Copernicus, and David Gans (who brought the geodetic tables to Latin Europe from Judeo-Arabic Spain, Neher 1986). Human-created things can go out of control and become destructive (Fukushima and Chernobyl, terminator seeds, industrial pollution, of which Frankenstein and Dr. Mabruse are also popular memes). But the story of the golem is not a call against the drive to create, only to try to avoid hubris in doing so, and thus learning to value the imperfections that allow infinite learning, feedback, responsibility, and responsiveness.

The golem's Jewish medieval history, as Gershom Scholem excavates, was primarily a mystical meditation protocol on animation and de-animation without (and even forbidden to have) practical purpose (beyond producing awe for God's or nature's power of creation). It could only be practiced by two scholars together, never by one alone. In earlier times, back to the creation of Adam, there are both tellurgic and pneumatic sources: adam is made of earth or clay (*adamah*) but also breath (*ruh, nefash*); Adam in one version was at first cosmically large stretching across the earth, and later reduced to human size, his breath only added at the very end of creation lest he claim to be a co-creator.

In Chinese one might call this *qui-shen*: "contractions-expansions," "outreach-return" of the winds and movements of the universe; or in miniature, more intimate, and everyday form, "ghosts and spirits" (Wang 2021).

The sixteenth century golem is said to be put away in the attic of the Altneu Synagogue of Prague next to the graveyard with 12,000 well-worn, crowded, overlapping, falling over, gravestones from 1439 to 1787, a veritable society of ghosts, traumatic memory, determined survival, or "living on" as Derrida might say, a site of *hauntogenesis* like many other such graveyards such as the great Bukit China in Malacca, the mummies in many Catholic catacombs and saints bones in altar-foundations of churches, or the hungry ghosts of the Vietnam War about which Heonik Kwon has written, including those of unidentified American or other foreign soldiers who also need care even if they were the enemy.

Genesis, the Greek word for Bereshit, the first word (and therefor the name) of the first book of the torah is *haunted* with the contradictions and alternative stories. It begins, after all, with *Bereshit* ("in the beginning"), with the *second, not the first* letter of the alphabet, shades of *emet/met* of the golem, but also shades of the separation of darkness from light, waters from the land, male from female, like, as Rahimi reminds us, the binary oppositions that make phonemes and thus spoken words, speech, *parole*. Not only are there two stories of Eve, one of the rib and one of full equality with Adam, not to mention Lilith; but there are also two stories of Adam, one a cosmogonic telluric giant of clay (Gen 1:24 "Let the earth bring forth living soul"), the other a pneuma (*neshumah*) blown into him. And all is shadowed or haunted by, infinite interpretations, partially collected in the talmud, the midrashim, and the agada, continuing into present day debates. Interpretive methods were generated in the "Babylonia" of the Persian Empire (today's southern Iraq), along with the contemporaneous and consociate interpretive traditions of Islam, disciplined by inductively established rules of logic and rhetoric, and by translations from the Greek disciplines of logic, rhetoric, and poetics.

Other perennial narrations, chasing present time rather than origins, Rahimi reminds us, are to be found in Shakespeare (*Hamlet*, three versions) and Goethe (*Faust*, and the predecessors from which Faust is drawn: the alchemist Johann Georg Faust, the playwright Christopher Marlowe,

Hrolf Kraki, the legend of Amieth in the thirteenth-century
m, and the tragic dramas of melancholy and insanity of the
century). In *Hamlet* time is over-anticipated, and in *Faust* it
comes indebted.

Hauntology, as Derrida introduces it to us in 1994, is a French hom-
onym for ontology that is the undoing of all ontology, all singularities, all
claims of singular origins, of singular sovereignties, of the unified self, and
of European philosophy as a restricted language game. Behind every claim
of "how things are" lie shadows, ghosts, temporary suppressions of alternatives and contestations in the rich possibilities of life, history, politics,
justice, and desire. The word comes from Old German via Old French. A
haunt is a place one frequents, a *Heim* or home, hence the importance of
the *unheimlich*, that which seems familiar, but not quite, the uncanny.

The uncanny is often located in dream, but today is increasingly experi-
mented with in future horizons: in English electronic music, in the
"uncanny valley" in the theater of robotics, and in future thinking art
works using generative algorithms and simulators. Unlike in the restricted
language game of Greek-based European philosophy where ontology in
the singular referred to the grounds of being (a challenging concept in
languages without a copula), computer scientists have introduced us to
plural ontologies, composed in object-oriented languages (like Java script).
Objects or protocols or machine instructions are given a cover term,
allowing them to be moved about as units without having to rewrite the
code each time. Ontologies are created by command lines. As computer
algorithms begin to drive more and more of our world, will this create a
flat world without shadows or ghosts, even as computer programs are built
up over generations with updates and patches and rewrites, and these can
create their own glitches, bugs, mis-directions, and openings for hackers,
and perhaps alternatives that are not washed out by redundancies, or fixed
by new generations of forensic mathematicians.

Might a primary solution to injustice and bias in the use of algorithms
be to have them written by the communities they are intended to help,
rather than by universality/ objectivity obsessed computer scientists, not
just so-called open source, or even free software. Does hauntology have a
place (or even a role in creating) future imaginaries, and what is the syntax
of that?

injustice and corruption, instead marshaling those things as evidence of a foreclosed world.

It is this jouissance and the resumption of the processes of democratization and pluralism, longed for in hauntology—including its engagements with the Real, and its surfacing of affects that seem to be signals from an emerging future—that is continued today in the electronic arts but also in a growing mood of active decolonial movements and insistence on restoring the commons, ecological sustainability, public goods, and community solidarities.

Hito Steyerl: Future Hauntologies, and the Challenges of Buen Vivir (Sumak Kawsay)

Change the shadow and then the object will change.
—Hito Steyerl, "Decolonize the Digital Sphere and Transition it Towards the Commons" (MIT, 2021)

Rahimi ends with a nod to the emergent cyber worlds of internet and virtual reality, new forms of power relations depending less on information than on simulacra: big data sets mined by machine learning algorithms, accelerated visual and sonic impressions, deep fakes in swarming circulation, memes that become data attractors and aggregators (collecting sentiments), networks (and data storage) hosting ghosts and revenants and doubles or multiples of ourselves, beyond explainability, but knowing (nudging, seducing, enticing) ourselves better than we ourselves ever can, hidden in plain sight but coded, embedded, encrypted, and flying by in signaling beyond the capacities of human senses. We are thus recruited also into the gamification of reality, the destabilization of time with proliferating apps ever forcing us into missing one another, the juxtapositions of increasingly inequalities, and above all, the further loosening of any links between the two meanings of "representation" in art and politics.

If one asks an Artificial Intelligence the old scholastic question, how many angels can dance on the head of a pin, as Hito Steyerl says she did (2019a), the answer it calculated, as did a friend, physicist of quantum entanglements, was 8.67 times ten to the 49th power. This assumes the angels dance at slightly less than the speed of light, because at any slower speed they will collapse into a black hole. Angels after all are pure intelligence or pure light. So if you ask an easier question such as, "does AI have a shadow?", the AI machine might say that angels don't have shadows. Still, says Steyerl, while we don't know what an AI is, the shadow of AI is already visible. (One of the key dilemmas of machine learning algorithms is that they are opaque to human intelligence. We can put them in motion and we can see what their outputs are, but mostly not how they get there.). The AI shadow moving ahead of our understanding is what we call "modeling" or "gaming". So the real question is not a quantitative one (i.e. about how many angels) but the nature of the dance or choreography. And one of the key features is about making things disappear and reappear, and often fragmenting time in the process.

And yet one of the key affordances of AI being utilized by scientists and artists alike is the self-generating ability to expand into the future, for instance using GANS technology (generative adversarial networks), a more sophisticated version of what used to be called A-Life or cellular automata (John H. Conway's 1970 *Game of Life*) and neural networks. Steyerl trains neural networks to extend images of flowers and plants, sometimes producing beautiful light sculptures. But primarily she is interested in whether one can grow a different kind of space (a latent or virtual space of potentialities), and then if one might be able to extend the growing of space to the physical world. Further, could one make the growing of spaces do some social justice work and help us toward new decolonized commons (as in her Free Plots/Pots project described below), or what in indigenous resistance and constitutional movements in the Andean countries of Bolivia, Columbia, and Ecuador is called in Quechua *sumak kawsay* or in Spanish *buen vivir* (creating the good life) in contrast to the production of waste and inequality by runaway capitalism.

How do we get there? One of Steyerl's recent projects, *Free Plots/Pots* is a standing riposte to the spread of Free Ports (and other invisibilizations of the infrastructure such as ports that no longer are open to citizen inspection and conviviality but are outside cities in gated, securitized spaces). One of Steyerl's videos was sold by her Paris gallerist for a sizeable sum to a French Art Foundation, and as she looked at the invoice, she was startled to see that the Foundation is incorporated within Geneva's Freeport (it is not the only such art foundation to be so incorporated). Made uncomfortable by this vehicle of tax evasion, avoiding paying taxes on artworks and thereby withholding funds from the French health care and cultural institution systems, Steyerl reinvested the money in two tons of composted horse manure which she donated to a community garden in

Berlin, providing them also Freeport shaped planters. The community garden is tended and *grown* by middle aged immigrant ladies, who plant beans that remind them of those from their homeland in Panama. The project has iterations in Spanish Harlem with immigrants from Puerto Rico, in Park Dale (Toronto), Amsterdam, and Luxembourg, all in community garden sites squeezed by gentrification Steyerl 2019a, b, c and 2021.

Taking pictures of the plants and supplementing them with an Oxford University flower data set, Steyerl trained another neural network to grow what she calls her own latent space of Free Plots, a probability space of all possible permutations of flowers grown in the Free Plots up to now. She discovered in so doing a layer of irises which she suggests might allude to, or in moebius strip fashion, return us to the Iris Data Set, devised by English statistician and eugenicist Ronald A. Fisher, that is still used to train students in the statistics for machine vision (and was critical to the development of socio-biology that reduced evolutionary models to selfish gene selection). Steyerl pushes this a bit further by saying this makes her think that Fisher's irises are stand-ins for human skulls, that "if one can discriminate flower species by superficial measurements" (his categories are things like petal size), "then one can also prove the existence of so-called races by just looking at people or measuring skulls or other visual criteria." The longer the process of growing flowers in Free Plots continues, she suggests, "we will essentially replace the standard academic Oxford data set with our own vernacular home grown flowers." But more importantly, the process is also one of growing physical spaces, which "compost" the Freeport-art-money world and constitute artificial territories elevated in *mobile* planters for urban community use. Moreover, she says, this is ideologically the extreme opposite of any kind of blood and soil idea of territory. And although ideas of organic agriculture and alternative ecologies are (and were in the past) captured by the right wing, this is not a *given*, not a *datum* (something "given") but a *factum* (something humanly made), and thus constitutes a different notion of truth and of territories, one dependent on the social activities of making by middle aged migrant ladies, growing their own "social spaces and community, with a certain autonomy and food sovereignty attached to it." The community gardens and Free Plots are spaces for story-telling, some of which Steyerl records and then plays from the Free Planters, but more important is their signifying of a social kind of photosynthesis: just as sunlight provides the "Power Plant" for life on earth processed by plants in photosynthesis, so too the Power Planters are social generators.

As the next step, since the money from the Freeport has run out, and new revenues are needed, she is devising a series of new "artworlds for compostation," or composting, via a blockchain Fintech device, perhaps using the cheese cryptocurrencies devised with a friend in Spain who owns sheep (shades of the "carbon coin" in Kim Stanley Robinson's *Ministry for the Future*, 2020) with which he speculates one could re-engineer the banking system to incentivize global climate warming reversal. Or perhaps Steyerl will use NTFs (non-fungible tokens) much talked about for selling in digital art markets. (NTFs exist in the Ethereum blockchain. You can store extra information so that when an artwork is downloaded not only does it operate as an authenticity certificate, but has extra value, and at each subsequent sale, the artist gets a percentage.)

But to return to the important issue of haunting and disappearance and return, and not only as speculative bubbles in the financial markets or gentrification as the displacement and disappearance of the poor, there is the more general problem of creative destruction which Steyerl explores in pieces called *The Language of Broken Glass* (2019), *Factory of the Sun* (2015), *How Not to Be Seen* (2013), and two videos about her childhood friend Andrea Wolf (*November*, and *Lovely Andrea*). As 17-year-olds, they used super-8 video to "shoot" feminist martial arts films; in 1988 Andrea ("Ronahi"), a sociologist writing a book on the PKK (the Kurdish guerilla party), was killed with 40 others in Çatak, southeast of Van, Turkey, in what Steyerl calls an "extra-judicial killing" by Turkish army forces, ironically enough, using guns from Germany. Asked about dealing with grief in her films, Steyerl, twenty years later, says that in the films Andrea is an imaginary figure albeit based on a real person, represented on a poster as a martyr. How does that relate to the fact that they made all these martial arts films together? But yes, the figure of Andrea follows Steyerl throughout her work, including an anime figure in Factory of the Sun. The question of what happened in 1988 catalyzed many other inquiries, and she gives a version of Freud's mourning and melancholia: "it is about not allowing grief to just take hold of yourself but just trying to transform it into lots of other situations." It is similar to the process of composting the Freeport into Free Plots. The ideas of energy (sunlight, photosynthesis, catalyst or catalyzing) and material realities constantly reforming and composting each other through acceleration and slowing are continuities in Steyerl's speculative re-imaging (in video) and re-imaging (in text) the potentialities of the world within which we are embedded, framed, degraded, and transformed, like poor images that gain circulatory power as they lose resolution, and can be passed from person to person, and node to node, and images that walk through screens to into reality Steyerl 2009, 2013a, b, 2016a, b.

Language of Broken Glass (2019), with its powerful title alluding to the Night of Broken Glass or *Kristalnacht* in November 1938) juxtaposes engineers in Cambridge, England, smashing thousands of windows — in order to train their AI to recognize the sound of breaking windows to put in home security devices to automatically alert the police — with community activists in New Jersey painting boarded up windows in a blighted area. Extrapolating and projecting the proliferation of such devices (also ring video home security devices that surveil the area in front of the door) Steyerl imagines market "win-win" incentives leading to a haunted ecology of increasing inequalities, defunding of services including police in favor of private militias to protect gated communities, or what she calls a luxury version of a war zone.

Factory of the Sun, picks up on the photosynthesis thread, and was inspired partly by Donna Haraway's, "our machines are made of pure sunlight" coding all information as well as human pain; partly by high frequency stock market trading and a faux report from CERN that they had made a particle accelerate beyond the speed of light (it was a loose cable); and partly by the lives of Julia and her brother, the dancer, TSC who appear in the film reprising some of their biographies. The video explores the technologies of motion capture, virtual reality 3600 video immersive media, and bubble vision, updating the Holodeck 3-D technology in Star Trek; and thereby attempts to "materialize" alternative worlds by animating futures with speculative visual technology experiments (Steyerl 2016, 2017, 2018). Real lives intertwine, not only with the actors, but also with the Ukrainians who worked on the postproduction animation. The video, in part, is set in a labor camp and Stalin's head explodes when shot by Julia, an effect that takes a lot of labor to pre-break it, but the head is cheap to buy on the Internet. Uncannily, its postproduction by Ukrainians in Karkov is being done under the shadow of the Russian invasion from the east. The Ukrainians are good both at rendering tanks as well as, for European clients, luxury hotels, malls, and gated communities (they actually look like Singapore more than Europe). *Factory of the Sun* is set in a motion capture studio (a labor camp of sorts in which everything is lighted and visible) and uses motion-movement-detection [MMD], staging the notion of "operational images," images made to be legible to machines more than to humans. But that shows how our sense of realism is increasingly gamified both visually and through the fact that everything collapses into a number, the score, that you achieve by your actions or inactions, whether you know it or not (credit scores for instance, or China's efforts at rolling out social credit scores). Like Haroun Farocki (from whom she takes the term "operational images", with its dual use in war targeting and post-traumatic stress disorder therapy) and Xu Bin's *Dragonfly Eyes* (a film and narrative composed completely with surveillance images), Steyerl in *How Not to Be Seen* (partly a tribute to a Monty Python piece from 1970) plays with how to disappear into the image, achieving invisibility even as one is being surveilled and monitored. The dark underside of this playful game, however, is not merely the gamification of remote control targeting from drones, but as a voice-over says,

> in the decade of the digital revolution 170,000 people disappear: disappeared people are annihilated, eliminated, irradicated, deleted, dispensed with, filtered, processed, selected, separated, wiped out. Invisible people retreat into 3-D animation, they hold the vectors of the nation to keep the picture together, they re-emerge as pixels, they merge into a world made of images.

As these lines are said, women in black burkas twirl on a chessboard-like platform in a desert. Steyerl comments:

> It's been that way for quite a while, but I think now, not only images, but all kinds of information are mostly made for machines by machines and they are coded in a way that is inaccessible to human senses altogether. So basically we live within this kind of chaos of signals zipping by which are absolutely inaccessible to human senses, so that basically most everything that could potentially be visible is completely removed from the reach of human senses … eyes or ears are not able to sense most relevant things anymore.

And yet, as Steyerl points out, while we like to think everything is monitored, there are vast unmonitored spaces. An airliner she notes can just disappear; there are spaces in Google Earth and Google Maps that are blank, just not there, impossible to access. There are over-monitored spaces and under-monitored ones. And our task is to grow the social spaces, the spaces that can flourish outside digital platforms formatted and owned by capitalist corporations and the military-art-complex. The international artworld of Biennales and fossil fuel flying around the world for shows has come to an end, she predicts. Interestingly, like Mark Fisher she has a date, his was 1985, hers is 2016, when the world began to change. "Progressive international art" needs to shift, she suggests, to both urban localities and to more rural and less populated areas, the latter for democratic decentralization, the former because cities have become themselves internationally diverse, and there is less need to network elsewhere, more need to build connections among citizens locally ("just go out, look around, say 'hello'").

There are prototypes she says for the detaching, de-colonizing, of digital platforms. Best known perhaps is the one led by Francesca Bria in Barcelona to municipalize data services and administer it through cooperatives. Politically more expansive is the constitutional drive in the Andean countries for *sumak kawsay* (the good life) in Quechua and *buen vivir* in Spanish and for "pluri-culturalism," terms which have been inserted into the Constitutions of Bolivia, Ecuador, and Columbia as counter-slogans and critique against extractive capitalism and neoliberal "development" plans (which usually involve the defunding of human services, education, health care, or their privatization for profit at the expense of the poor). And it is grounded in what are thought of as ancestral indigenous knowledges, metaphorized and spoken of as living in concert, dialogue, and engagement with the spirits of the non-human world. This idiom competes for political hegemony in designing public goods and public spaces, and in protecting the environment. It acts as a check on half-way measures of hegemonic power structures that tout benevolence in the form of philanthropy (instead of social infrastructure), socially responsible corporate investments (while protecting profits), providing individual choice (instead of protection of community and social solidarity), individual insurance plans (instead of public health).

Whether or not the spirit worlds are hauntological may be a matter of opinion, but they have to do with the familiar haunts of living with nature, ecological forces, and symbiosis; they are guided and reinforced by rituals that engage the spirit worlds, often in healthier ways than prosperity religions, witch-hunts, or other us-them panics. Efforts to decolonize the media have been on-going as well both in the struggle for use of Linux and open software rather than large corporate systems (Microsoft) in government bureaucracies in various parts of Latin America, including Peru. Among the most interesting of the struggles to see how one might integrate *sumak kawsay* and *public health* is an on-going dialogue in Columbia with competing understandings not just of health care but of local autonomy and sovereignty over future lives. This is not just a matter of slogans, and certainly not simple-minded nostalgia for the past, but hard efforts to work across practicalities, and social justice, what Lyotard meant perhaps by "just gaming" (gaming for justice, just play as mode of learning) and Harocki by "Serious Games." The power of such revival of another way of thinking (which themselves are plural) may in the case of biology have an interface with new interests in signaling among trees, concern with ghost species (which continue to exist but are past the point of population collapse), or even the reanimation of extinct species (as in the Siberian project to use mammoth DNA to breed elephants that can withstand extreme cold and help restore the softening tundra bogs, before they release vast amounts of methane). AI systems are often replacements by cost-cutting anti-conservation governments for on-the ground experimental knowledge, and such rapprochement with people who want to live in situ as stewards of the earth and its hauntologies could be invaluable.

Conclusion: Bereshit, Catacoustics, and Shadows

It is uncanny (scarily similar, unnervingly different) how the three historical horizons with their different affordances and takes, sketched above, deal differently with time, space, projection, melancholy-grief, socialities, and assumptions of machine, human and biological capacities. From the *Nachträglichkeit* (belated, triggered) repression-returns of Hauntology in the Freudian-Lacanian era to the layering, sampling, rhythm disruptions and reconstructions of the sonic Hauntology in the 1980s–2010s, to the catalyzing and self-generating growth of new social processes to underpin our expanding electronic arts and bioarts understandings of worlds where the present is an unstable construct, realism is never natural but labored and peopled, and where *datum* and *factum* oscillate making appearances disappear and return otherwise in the uncanny, and the Real.

References

Derrida, J. (1994). *Specters of Marx: The State of the Debt, the Work of Mourning, and the New International.* Trans. P. Kamuf. Routledge.

Fisher, M. (2014). *Ghosts of My Life: Writings on Depression, Hauntology and Lost Futures.* John Hunt Publishing.

Fisher, M. (2018). *K-Punk: The Collected and Unpublished Writings of Mark Fisher (2004–16)*. Repeater Books.

Neher, A. (1986). *Jewish Thought and the Scientific Revolution of the Sixteenth Century: David Gans, 1541–1613, and His Times*. Oxford University Press.

Robinson, K. S. (2020). *The Ministry for the Future*. Little, Brown Book Group.

Ronell, A. (2002). *Stupidity*. University of Illinois Press.

Scholem, G. G. (1965). *On the Kabbalah and Its Symbolism*. Routledge and Kegan Paul.

Steyerl, H. (2009). *In Defense of the Poor Image*. E-flux, No. 10, November. https://www.e-flux.com/journal/10/61362/in-defense-of-the-poor-image/

Steyerl, H. (2013a). *I Dreamed a Dream: Politics in the Age of Mass Art Production*. Lecture, Former West Research Congress, Haus der Kulturen der West, Berlin.

Steyerl, H. (2013b). *The Photographic University: Photography and Political Agency?* Lecture, New School for Social Research, New York. https://www.youtube.com/watch?v=kqQ3UTWSmUc

Steyerl, H. (2013c). How Not to Be Seen: A Fucking Didactic Educational .Mov File. *Art Forum*. https://www.artforum.com/video/hito-steyerl-how-not-to-be-seen-a-fucking-didactic-educational-mov-file-2013-51651

Steyerl, H. (2015). *The Terror of Total Dasein*. Lecture as Part of Former West Public Editorial Meeting, Art and Labor after the End of Work, Museum of Modern Art, Warsaw. https://www.youtube.com/watch?v=SI0Mw7ASl3A

Steyerl, H. (2016). *What Is Contemporary Art? A Conversation with Hito Seyerl*. Museum of Contemporary Art. https://www.youtube.com/watch?v=sNW1PP-034Q

Steyerl, H. (2017 and 2018). *Bubble Vision*. The Serpentine Gallery, London (2017). University of Michigan Stamps School of Art and Design (2018). https://www.youtube.com/watch?v=T1Qhy0_PCjs

Steyerl, H. (2019a). *The Language of Broken Glass*. Haus der Kulturen der Welt, Berlin. https://www.youtube.com/watch?v=iyyM4vDg0xw

Steyerl, H. (2019b). *This Is the Future*. Artist's Talk at Art Gallery of Ontario. https://www.youtube.com/watch?v=ts-dNHeBtdQ

Steyerl, H. (2019c). *Power Plants, AI, and Music*. Serpentine Galleries, London. https://www.youtube.com/watch?v=1v08U5-B

Steyerl, H. (2021). Decolonize the Digital Sphere and Transition It Towards the Commons. Closing address at MIT List Visual Arts Center Max Wasserman Forum: Another World.

Wang, J. (2021). *Half Sound, Half Philosophy: Aesthetics, Politics and History of China's Sound Art*. Bloomsbury Academic.

INDEX[1]

[1] Note: Page numbers followed by 'n' refer to notes.

© The Author(s), under exclusive license to Springer Nature Switzerland AG 2021
S. Rahimi, *The Hauntology of Everyday Life*,
https://doi.org/10.1007/978-3-030-78992-3

97

CPSIA information can be obtained
at www.ICGtesting.com
Printed in the USA
BVHW012124220821
614973BV00002BA/45

9 783030 789916